Distributed in USA and Canada by:
J.B. Lippincott Company
East Washington Square
Philadelphia, PA 19105
USA

Distributed in Philippines/Guam, Middle East, Latin America and Africa by:
Harper & Row International
East Washington Square
Philadelphia, PA 19105
USA

Distributed in UK and Continental Europe by:
Harper & Row Ltd.
Middlesex House
34-42 Cleveland Street
London W1P 5FB
UK

Distributed in Australia and New Zealand by:
Harper & Row (Australasia) Pty Ltd.
P.O. Box 226
Artarmon, N.S.W. 2064
Australia

Distributed in Southeast Asia, Hong Kong, India and Pakistan by:
Harper & Row Publishers (Asia) Pte Ltd.
37 Jalan Pemimpin 02-01
Singapore 2057

Distributed in Japan by:
Igaku Shoin Ltd.
Tokyo International
P.O. Box 5063
Tokyo
Japan

Library of Congress Cataloging-in-Publication Data
Contact lens fitting.
   Bibliography: p.
   Includes index.
   1. Contact lenses.   2. Contact lenses—Atlases.
I. Weinstock, Frank J., 1933–
RE977.C6C5577   1989   617.7′523   88-21310
ISBN 0-397-44671-3

British Library Cataloguing in Publication Data
Contact lenses.
   1. Contact lenses
   1. Weinstock, Frank J.
   617.7′523
   ISBN 0-397-44671-3

Editor   Karen L. Dean
Art Director Jill Feltham
Illustrators Sue Ann Fung and Carol Kalafatic
Designer   Thomas Tedesco

Printed in Hong Kong by
Imago Publishing, Ltd.

FOREWORD

Why another book on contact lenses? Primarily because few contact lens books have been written by Ophthalmologists with the experience of these authors. Each author is an expert in his or her contact lens area. Gower publications is an expert in graphics, illustrations and photographic reproductions. The combined talents of the authors and the publisher result in the production of a high quality book which is in a class by itself.

The care of contact lens patients has reached somewhat of a crisis because, as the number of contact lens wearers has increased, the number of complications of contact lens wear has increased also. The serious complications must be managed by Ophthalmologists who also must play a significant role in their prevention by being familiar with the proper fitting and follow-up care of contact lenses. Their knowledge and involvement will be assisted considerably by reading practical books such as this one.

With limited instruction in the area of contact lenses available during residency training, this volume assumes great importance because both basic fitting of lenses and state of the art advances in contact lens technology are covered. This is especially significant with the increased interest of patients in contact lenses and with the advances which enable more patients than ever to obtain improved vision with contact lenses. Fitting lenses and coming to the meetings of the Contact Lense Association of Ophthalmologists (CLAO) will complete residents training so that the unfamiliarity of contact lenses will not interfere with their taking care of contact lens wearers.

I applaud Dr. Weinstock's interest and efforts in taking charge of the completion of this useful book which will be of great use to residents and Ophthalmologists in practice, as well as their office staffs.

R. Linsy Farris, M.D.
Professor of Clinical Ophthalmology
Edward S. Harkness Eye Institute of
Columbia-Presbyterian Medical Center,
New York

PREFACE

Large, small, steep, flat—these were the decisions to be made for contact lens fitting in the not too distant past when only one material—PMMA—was available for daily wear.

Modern technology has provided us with a plethora of materials and options in the exciting field of contact lenses, giving us lenses for daily or extended wear, disposable lenses, single vision, astigmatic, and bifocal lenses in soft, hard, or gas-permeable materials. Each may have specific indications, fitting techniques, care regimens, and potential complications.

For a period of time it appeared as if soft lenses would make rigid materials obsolete. In fact, many training programs have essentially ignored the entire field of rigid materials, concentrating only on soft lenses. A competent fitter must be knowledgeable about all the options available today. This includes the needs of the individual patient and characteristics of each type of lens.

The high degree of sophistication attained is not without problems for the fitter and for the patient. These problems include the basic decision of which lens to fit on which patient, how to fit and care for the chosen lens, and how to recognize specific problems such as poor vision, solution sensitivity, giant papillary conjunctivitis, and poorly fitting lenses.

Interpretation of fluorescein patterns and meticulous monitoring of the cornea and eye for changes and potential problems have restored much of the art and science to contact lens fitting. It is not possible to simply pick a lens from a chart, give it to the patients, and discharge the patient.

This book contains a wealth of up-to-date information which will be valuable to new fitters as well as the most experienced fitters and their office staffs. Each author presents the latest material in his or her area of expertise in his or her own words and style.

Frank J. Weinstock, M.D., F.A.C.S.
Canton, Ohio

CONTRIBUTORS

MARK BALLOW, M.D.
Eye Physician Associates
Hartford, Connecticut

PATRICK J. CAROLINE, C.O.T.
Director of Contact Lens Research
Estelle Doheny Eye Medical Clinic, Inc.
Los Angeles, California

PETER C. DONSHIK, M.D.
Eye Physician Associates
Hartford, Connecticut

JOHN B. FRANKLIN, M.D., F.A.C.S.
Hartford, Connecticut

MICHAEL HARRIS, M.D.
Livingston, New Jersey

RONALD HERSKOWITZ, O.D.
Vice President, Technical Affairs
Polymer Technology
Wilmington, Massachusetts

MICHAEL LEMP, M.D.
Georgetown University
Washington, D.C.

ANGELA E. LUISTRO, C.O.T.
Eye Physician Associates
Hartford, Connecticut

EZRA MAGUEN, M.D.
Cedars Sinai Medical Center
Los Angeles, California

LEROY MESHEL, M.D.
Director, Narcissus Medical Research Foundation
Daly City, California

CRAIG W. NORMAN, C.O.T., F.C.L.S.A.
Director, Contact Lens Section,
Department of Ophthalmology
South Bend Clinic
South Bend, Indiana

DIANN PINNER-RYAN, C.O.T.
Georgetown University
Washington, D.C.

JOSEPH W. SOPER, F.C.L.S.A.
Baylor College of Medicine
Houston, Texas

SHELDON WECHSLER, O.D.
Vistakon
Jacksonville, Florida

FRANK J. WEINSTOCK, M.D., F.A.C.S.
Northeastern Ohio Universities College of Medicine and
Ohio State University
Canton, Ohio

CONTENTS

vii

1
RIGID CONTACT LENSES —HARD AND GAS-PERMEABLE

JOHN B. FRANKLIN, M.D., F.A.C.S.,
FRANK J. WEINSTOCK, M.D., F.A.C.S.,
PATRICK J. CAROLINE, C. O. T.,
CRAIG W. NORMAN, C.O.T.

During the high point of soft contact lens (Fig. 1.1) popularity in the 1970s, many people predicted the demise of the rigid contact lens. For a number of years it appeared that the pessimists were going to prevail, but rigid lens fittings, especially the gaspermeable (RGP) fitting, increased by 50% in 1985, as compared to a 25% increase in soft lens fittings in the same year (1).

The rise in popularity of rigid contact lenses (Fig. 1.2) has been due to practitioner dissatisfaction with many undesirable features of soft contact lenses. For example, it has been noted that the vision obtainable with a rigid contact lens is often superior to the best vision obtainable with a soft contact lens. Some of the reasons for this observation are noted in Table 1.1.

Superior visual characteristics, durability, and cost effectiveness contribute to the increasing popularity of rigid contact lenses, which do not tear or tend to accumulate deposits in patients with dry eyes. Since they do not place the same hydration demands on the eye as soft lenses, they may provide better vision for patients in dry climates and environments.

In a recent telephone survey by one of us (JBF), most contact lens practitioners stated that they are no longer fitting rigid polymethylmethacrylate (PMMA) lenses ("hard" lenses) except for replacements or where the patient desires a hard PMMA lens for a specific reason such as cost. All special lens designs, including toric, bifocal, prism ballast, Soper cone, myoflange, and hyperflange, are available in gas-permeable materials. The rigid gas-permeable lenses may be ordered with a custom edge design and may be modified using standard velveteen and moleskin tools if a special polishing compound is used (2).

Reports in the literature by one of us [JBF (3)] and others have indicated that RGP lenses are suitable for extended wear. Some RGP lenses are approved by the FDA for extended wear.

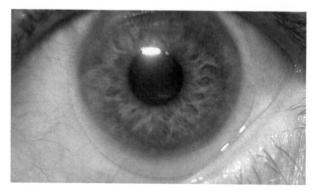

Fig. 1.1 *Soft contact lens.*

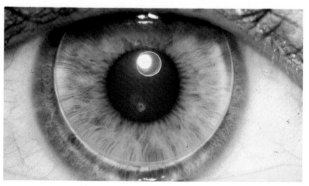

Fig. 1.2 *Rigid contact lens.*

Table 1.2 lists D_k values of some currently available materials. The higher values indicate greater oxygen permeability.

In addition to ease of fit and the ability to have lenses tinted (Fig. 1.3), other advantages of RGP lenses are summarized in Table 1.3. RGP lenses are indicated for visual correction when visual correction cannot be obtained with a soft lens, when soft

TABLE 1.1
VISUAL ADVANTAGES OF A RIGID LENS

1. Air/lens interface is fixed and rigid rather than undulant and soft.
2. Astigmatism up to 3 or 4 diopters may be filled in by tears on which the rigid lens rides.
3. Surface problems inherent to soft contact lenses are not found with the rigid lenses, thereby reducing light scatter and halos.
4. Because of higher oxygen transmissibility, rigid gas-permeable lenses may cause less corneal edema than soft lenses.

TABLE 1.2
D_K (FATT) VALUES OF RIGID GAS-PERMEABLE MATERIALS

Material	D_K (35°)
Polycon II	12.0
Boston IV	28.7
Paraperm EW	37.3
SGP II	39.0
Equalens	70.0

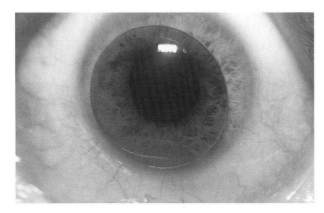

Fig. 1.3 *Tinted contact lens.*

TABLE 1.3
ADVANTAGES OF RIGID GAS-PERMEABLE LENSES (SUMMARY)

1. Ease of fit: Although it is best to use a specific trial lens set, some lenses may be fit with any standard trial set.
2. There are a variety of special lens designs available, e.g., toric, bifocal, myoflange, hyperflange, and prism ballast.
3. Practitioner modifiable.
4. Radiuscope verifiable.
5. Lensometer readable.
6. Visual advantages (see Table 1.1).
7. Extended wear option.
8. Tintable.
9. Durable.
10. Cost effective.
11. Use in drier eyes.

lenses are no longer tolerated in such conditions as giant papillary conjunctivitis, or when a patient desires a rigid lens for the reasons listed above.

One of the earliest noted great advantages to the use of soft contact lenses was the possibility of intermittent wear (e.g., going out to dinner on Saturday night). Although this is not recommended for hard contact lens wearers who must maintain a minimum wearing schedule, this intermittent use does not seem to be a problem for the patient with RGP lenses.

The overwearing syndrome of acute central corneal edema (Fig. 1.4) (namely, erosions due to corneal anoxia), which was well known to the contact lens practitioner of the 1960s and early 1970s, has largely disappeared with the advent of the soft contact lens. Although it may rarely occur with RGP or soft lenses, it is unusual.

Similarly, the hard lens inadvertent corneal molding with chronic changes in the corneal shape, as demonstrated by blurred keratometric mires and inability to wear glasses following lens removal (spectacle blur), has largely disappeared with soft and RGP lenses. When used for deliberate corneal molding in orthokeratology, the incidence of corneal erosions is decreased.

Hard contact lenses are contraindicated in poorly motivated patients, patients with poor compliance and poor hygiene, and patients with minimal refractive errors. Many fitters feel that athletes engaged in contact sports may do better with soft contact lenses than with RGP lenses since there is less likelihood of lens decentration with the larger soft lenses.

The chief disadvantage of the RGP lens is the lens sensation which is noticed by most patients initially. However, when soft contact lens wearers are switched over to RGP lenses, they

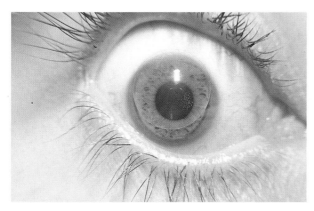

Fig. 1.4 *Contact lens keratopathy (overwearing).*

TABLE 1.4 PATIENT EVALUATION AND SELECTION CONSIDERATIONS
1. Sex
2. Age
3. Personal hygiene
4. Environmental needs
5. Occupational needs
6. Refractive considerations
7. Medical eye evaluation and examination

usually state that, after the initial adaption, there is no sensation difference noted between the two lenses.

A new contact lens, the Saturn, marries a rigid gas-permeable lens centrally to a peripheral soft contact lens skirt, with the aim of providing both soft contact lens comfort and rigid lens vision. This lens is expensive, difficult to fit and remove, and has a limited use as a problem-solving lens.

PATIENT EVALUATION AND SELECTION

The criteria given in Table 1.4 are evaluated. It is generally conceded that females are better contact lens candidates than males. Although there are no maximum or minimum age criteria for contact lens fitting for cosmetic use, children should be old enough to care for an item as delicate and expensive as a contact lens. As patients age, fitting myopic patients with contact lenses increases the accommodative demands and may precipitate the need for reading glasses in patients in their thirties and forties. The increased accommodative demand may have an adverse effect on esophorias or tropias (Figs. 1.5 and 1.6). Hyperopic

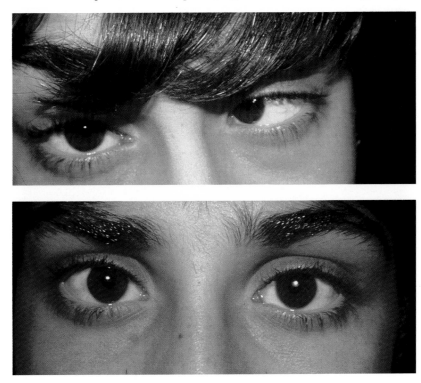

Fig. 1.5 *Accommodative esotropia (worsened with single-vision contact lenses).*

Fig. 1.6 *Accommodative esotropia (corrected with rigid multifocal contact lenses).*

corrections with contact lenses may weaken accommodative demands and worsen an exo-deviation.

A rapid scan of the patient's appearance (dirty fingernails and hands, etc.) may alert the practitioner to a person who will take less than ideal care of his or her contact lenses, thereby increasing the possibility of infection and complications. Medical eye conditions such as blepharitis should be evaluated and treated before fitting is undertaken.

Occupational exposure to dusty or dry environments (such as the workplace environments of entertainers or athletes) may have impact on lens selection. Refractive requirements such as astigmatism, the need for clearer vision than might be obtained with soft lenses, or bifocal needs must be considered.

FITTING RIGID LENSES

A complete evaluation of the patient, including refraction, corneal topography, and determination of the presence or absence of disease conditions and possible contraindications to contact lenses, is carried out.

After the decision to fit a contact lens has been made by the fitter and the patient, a choice of rigid hard or gas-permeable lens materials is made using the criteria in Table 1.5.

TABLE 1.5
SELECTION CRITERIA FOR RIGID HARD OR GAS-PERMEABLE LENSES

1. Astigmatism over 1.00 diopters
2. Small palpebral fissures
3. Small corneal diameters
4. Special design requirements:
   Keratoconus
   Bifocal (also available in soft)
   Toric (also available in soft)
   Iris painted (also available in soft)
   Occluder (also available in soft)

5. Extended wear in patient with astigmatism (limited FDA approval as of April 1988)
6. Intolerance to soft lenses or solutions
7. Patient who developed giant papillary conjunctivitis while wearing soft lenses
8. Intermittent wear requirements

TERMINOLOGY

The contact lens rests on the cornea and is described by the variables shown in Fig. 1.7. The *base curve* is the posterior surface curve (radius) of the lens and is measured in millimeters or converted to diopters. This corresponds to the posterior optical zone and is related to the corneal curvature (also measured in millimeters or diopters), which is measured with a keratometer (e.g., base curve 7.50 mm = 45.00 diopters).

The *power* or strength of the lens is measured (in diopters) with the lensometer and is related to the refraction of the patient (e.g., contact lens power = −6.00 diopters).

The *diameter* of the lens and of the *optical zone* (O.Z.) is measured in millimeters (e.g., diameter = 9.2 mm, O.Z. = 7.8 mm). Too small a diameter or optical zone may cause distortion when the edge is seen.

The *center thickness* (C.T.) is measured in millimeters at the geometric center of the lens and must be correct to prevent flexure and to allow oxygen flux through the lens (e.g., C.T. = 0.12 mm).

Figure 1.8 demonstrates that the *peripheral curve* is the flattest curve at the periphery of the lens, whereas the *secondary* or *intermediate curve* is adjacent to and flatter than the base curve. These curves allow a smooth fit at the periphery of the cornea,

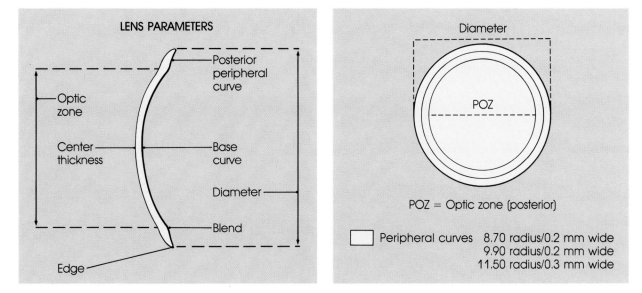

Fig. 1.7 *Lens parameters.*

Fig. 1.8 *Peripheral curves and optic zone.*

assist in oxygen transmission at the corneal surface, and support a tear meniscus at the edge of the lens which aids in lens centration (e.g., peripheral curves: 8.70 radius/0.2 mm wide, 11.50 mm radius/0.3 mm wide) (Fig. 1.8).

Lenses are usually spherical, with every meridian having the same radius of curvature. The radius of curvature of the front surface is determined by the lens manufacturer. With residual astigmatic corrections, a toric front surface may be used (e.g., spectacle prescription = 1.50 diopters − 1.75 cx 180°, keratometry = 44.00 × 180° and 44.75 × 90°). The residual astigmatism is 1.00 diopters. Back-surface toricity may be necessary for control of rotation and centering with higher degrees of corneal astigmatism. *Bi-toric* lenses have a toric anterior and

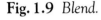

Fig. 1.9 *Blend.*

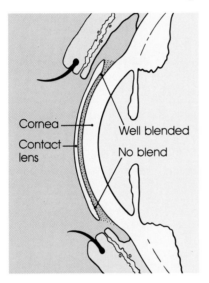

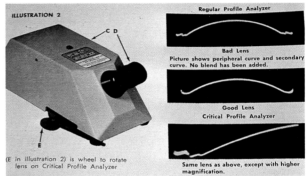

Fig. 1.10 *Profile analyzer, with examples of good and bad peripheral curve blending.*

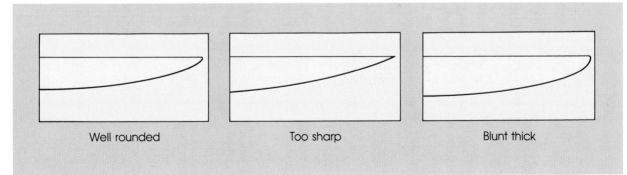

Fig. 1.11 *Edge design.*

posterior surface to improve positioning and correct residual astigmatism in patients with high degrees of corneal astigmatism.

The junction area between the peripheral curves should have a smooth *blend* for best comfort (Fig. 1.9). This area is evaluated with the profile analyzer (Fig. 1.10), an indispensable tool for evaluation and correction of uncomfortable lenses. The edge should be smooth (Fig. 1.11).

In order to thin a lens edge with a high prescription, a plus lens carrier design (*hyperflange*) may be used (Figs. 1.12 and 1.13). It may be necessary to use the minus carrier design (*myoflange*) to increase the edge thickness to improve the centration of a low-riding lens (Fig. 1.14).

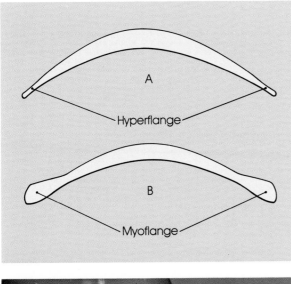

Fig. 1.12 *Hyperflange and myoflange design. The plus lens carrier design, often referred to as a hyperflange (A), thins the lens edge; the minus carrier design, known as a myoflange (B), increases edge thickness to aid a low-riding lens to center better.*

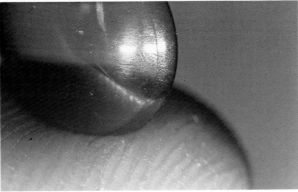

Fig. 1.13 *Soper hyperflange contact lens.*

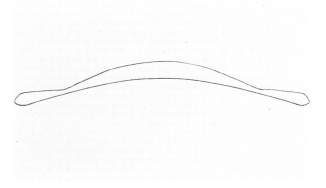

Fig. 1.14 *Soper myoflange design.*

Prism ballast (Fig. 1.15) increases the thickness and weight of a lens for stabilization or allows the lower lid to force the lens upward during downgaze with some bifocal lens designs. Adding *truncation* (Fig. 1.16) will assist in stabilization of the low-riding lens, which may slip beneath the lower lid.

The *lenticular* design is used to decrease the overall lens mass for better centering by increasing or decreasing the edge thickness of the lens.

Keratometry involves the use of a manual (Figs. 1.17 and 1.18) or automated (Fig. 1.19) keratometer to measure the curvature (in diopters) of the front surface of the cornea. The astigmatism is the difference between two readings 90° apart. Usually, minus cylinder notations are used (e.g., horizontal = 42.00 diopters, vertical = 44.00 diopters × 180). *With-the-rule* astigmatism has the greater power in the vertical axis (e.g., H = 42.00, V = 44.00 × 90), whereas *against-the-rule* astigmatism has the greater power in the horizontal meridian (e.g., H = 44.00, V = 42.00 × 180).

Prior to the advent of RGP materials, hard lenses were originally fit by ordering a lens based on the refraction and keratometric readings, usually 0.25 diopter steeper than the flattest K reading, with some modification for the corneal astigmatism.

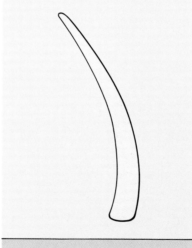

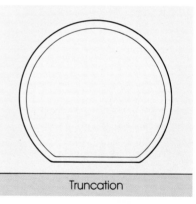

Truncation

Fig. 1.15 *Prism ballast. It may be necessary to increase the thickness, and consequently the weight of a lens to stabilize the lens position, aiding in meridional orientation. This increased lens thickness can also allow the lower lid to force the lens upward during downgaze, such as in some types of bifocal contact lenses.*

Prism ballast

Fig. 1.16 *Truncation. Sometimes, after prism ballast has been added to a lens, the lens rides too low, slipping underneath the lower lid, thus not aiding the lens positioning. If this occurs, the inferior portion of the lens can be removed or truncated to assist in stabilization.*

The fitter usually had a preferred size. In the earlier years, large flat lenses ranging in size from 9.0 to 10.0 mm were used. Later on, smaller, steeper lenses were used, usually 8.5–8.7 mm in size. After the examination was carried out, the lens was ordered and delivered to the patient at another visit.

In the search for efficiency, the use of fitting and inventory (Fig. 1.20) sets enabled the evaluation and dispensing of lenses to be carried out on the initial visit. A lens from the fitting set is placed on the eye and is evaluated by slit-lamp observation and refraction. A lens is then taken from the inventory and is dispensed to the patient with instruction as to insertion, removal, wearing routine, and care. In addition to eliminating a second visit, the inventory is of great help in replacing damaged and lost lenses. The hard lens inventory may run from hundreds

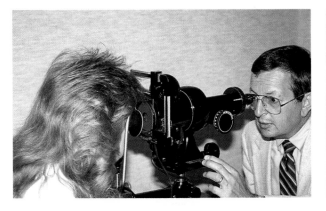

Fig. 1.17 *Manual keratometer with Soper topogometer.*

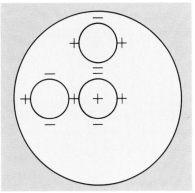

Fig. 1.18 *Mires on cornea as seen through the manual Bausch & Lomb keratometer.*

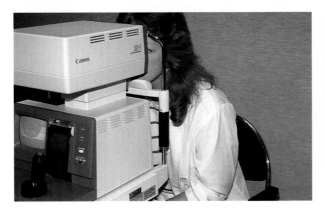

Fig. 1.19 *Automated keratometer.*

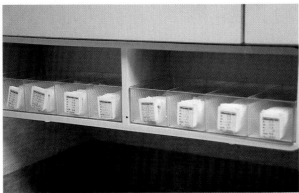

Fig. 1.20 *Inventory lenses.*

to thousands of lenses and usually pays for itself as a result of the increased efficiency.

With the plethora of RGP materials, it is most satisfactory to use a fitting set, in the material to be used, from the individual company that will manufacture the lens. Inventory fitting may also be used with RGP materials in spite of their higher cost. This will, of course, limit the fitter to one or two materials. Fitting too many types of lenses, in addition to the cost of fitting sets and inventories, may be quite confusing to the fitter.

It is desirable to have a light tint incorporated in contact lenses to make the lenses more visible when they are off of the eye. The tints usually do not adversely affect color or night vision. If the tint is too dark (e.g., number 3 tint), twilight and night driving may become dangerous.

After the ocular examination, keratometry and refraction (Fig. 1.21) are carried out and the decision is made to fit an RGP lens; the fitting is carried out by choosing a lens from the fitting set and placing it on the eye according to the formula in Table 1.6. This is best done without a topical anesthetic so that the patient is aware of what the sensation should be. In a small number of sensitive patients, excess tearing will require the use of a drop of topical anesthetic for an adequate evaluation of the fit.

For a myopic patient a diagnostic set may be:

DIAMETER	POWER	BASE CURVE RANGE (IN 0.50-DIOPTER STEPS)
9.2 mm	−3.00 diopters	40.00 diopters (8.44 mm) to 47.00 diopters (7.18 mm)

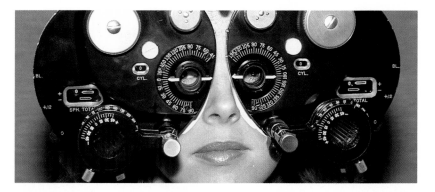

Fig. 1.21 *Phoropter for refraction (over-refraction of some contact lenses may require the use of individual lenses in a trial frame).*

RIGID CONTACT LENSES

Additional diameters of 8.7 mm and 9.7 mm are helpful.

EXAMPLE: $K = 42.75/44.25 \times 90$

DIAGNOSTIC LENS: BC, 43.00 diopters (7.85 mm);
power, -3.00 diopters; diameter, 9.2 mm.

The lens should position superiorly, with the upper edge of the lens approaching the superior limbus and remaining covered by the lid during the blink (Figs. 1.22 and 1.23). A more central

TABLE 1.6
CORNEAL ASTIGMATISM WITH RESPECT TO CORNEAL ASTIGMATISM FACTOR

Amount of Corneal Astigmatism (in diopters)	Corneal Astigmatism Factor (with respect to the flattest K)		
	9.7 mm	9.2 mm	8.7 mm
0.00–0.50	0.50 flatter	0.25 flatter	On flat K
0.75–1.25	0.25 flatter	On flat K	0.25 steeper
1.50–2.00	On flat K	0.25 steeper	0.50 steeper
2.25–2.75	0.25 steeper	0.50 steeper	0.75 steeper
3.00–3.50	0.50 steeper	0.75 steeper	1.00 steeper

The corneal astigmatism values that are "flatter" than the flattest K measurement are *subtracted* from the flat K; the values that are "steeper" are *added* to the flat K.

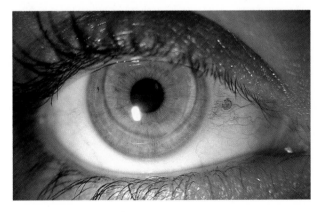

Fig. 1.22 *Well-fitting RGP contact lens.*

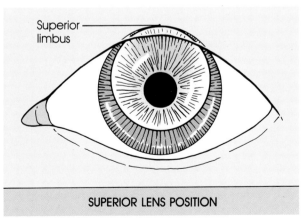

Superior limbus

SUPERIOR LENS POSITION

Fig. 1.23 *Superior lens position.*

fit is often acceptable also (Fig. 1.24). The lens should be large enough to cover the pupil in dim illumination and should move $1-1\frac{1}{2}$ mm with each blink (Fig. 1.25).

If the lens positions too low (Fig. 1.26), replace it with a lens that is 0.25–0.50 diopter (0.05–0.10 mm) flatter, which will

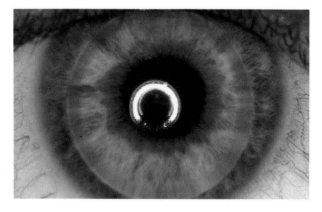

Fig. 1.24 *Central-fitting RGP contact lens.*

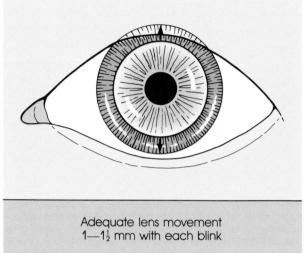

Adequate lens movement
$1-1\frac{1}{2}$ mm with each blink

Fig. 1.25 *Adequate lens movement $1-1\frac{1}{2}$ mm with each blink.*

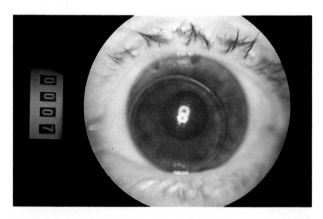

Fig. 1.26 *Low-riding contact lens.*

allow the lid to pull the lens up. The effect may be intensified by using a larger-diameter lens, as shown in Fig. 1.27.

The fluorescein pattern should demonstrate minimal apical clearance and is best seen with the blue filter on the slit lamp (Figs. 1.28 and 1.29). A steep lens will show excessive apical

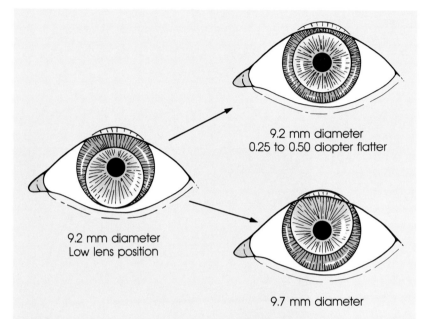

Fig. 1.27 *Management of low lens positioning.*

9.2 mm diameter
0.25 to 0.50 diopter flatter

9.2 mm diameter
Low lens position

9.7 mm diameter

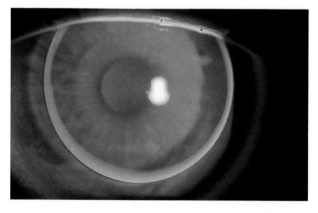

Fig. 1.28 *Fluorescein pattern of slight apical clearance.*

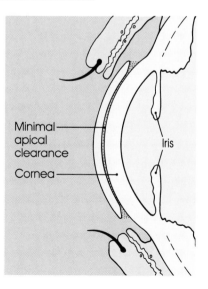

Minimal apical clearance

Cornea

Iris

Fig. 1.29 *Minimal apical clearance or alignment pattern.*

clearance and midperipheral touch (Figs. 1.30 and 1.31).

The lens power is directly obtained by refracting over the diagnostic lens and adding the two powers. If a mathematical formula is used the vertex distance tables must be consulted in powers over 5.00 diopters and compensation for the difference between the two *K* readings must be made. When the base curve is steeper than the flat *K*, a plus tear lens is created behind the lens requiring the addition of minus power equal to the difference between the base curve and the flat *K* [mnemonic is SAM (steeper—add minus)] (Fig. 1.32).

When fit on *K*, the tear lens power is zero and requires no compensation (Fig. 1.33).

With a flatter than *K* base curve, a minus tear lens is created

Fig. 1.30 *Tight (steep) contact lens—fluorescein pattern.*

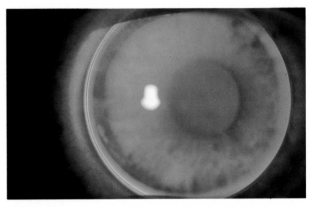

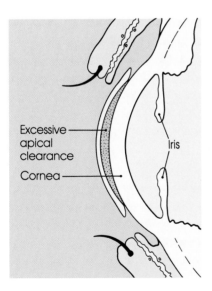

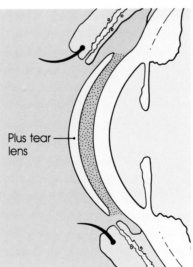

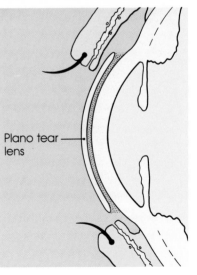

Fig. 1.31 *Steep lens/cornea relationship.*

Fig. 1.32 *Plus tear lens SAM (steeper—add minus).*

Fig. 1.33 *Plano tear lens.*

RIGID CONTACT LENSES

which requires the addition of plus power equal to the difference between the flat *K* and the base curve [mnemonic is FAP (flatter—add plus)] (Fig. 1.34).

For hyperopic fitting a diagnostic fitting set may be:

DIAMETER	POWER	RANGE OF BASE CURVES (0.50-DIOPTER STEPS)	DESIGN
8.7 mm	+ 3.00 diopters	42.00 diopters (8.04 mm) to 47.00 diopters (7.18 mm)	Single cut
9.2 mm	+ 3.00 diopters	40.00 diopters (8.44 mm) to 46.00 diopters (7.34 mm)	Lenticular

Start with an 8.7-mm single-cut diagnostic lens of the base curve indicated above and evaluate the position of the lens. If the lens positions centrally or slightly low, go to a smaller diameter, usually no less than 8.5 mm. If this is not effective, change to a larger lens (9.2 mm) with a lenticular design, remembering to flatten the base curve when going to a larger diameter (Fig. 1.35). The fluorescein pattern should show a slight apical clearance or apical alignment pattern (Fig. 1.28).

When the positioning is correct, refract over the lens in order to obtain the correct power.

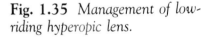

Fig. 1.35 *Management of low-riding hyperopic lens.*

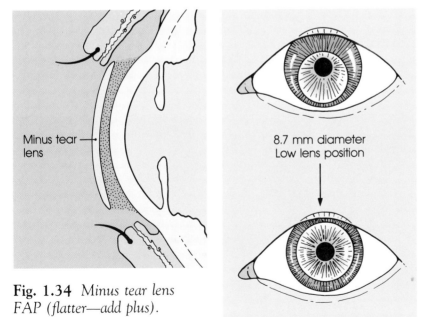

Fig. 1.34 *Minus tear lens FAP (flatter—add plus).*

Minus tear lens

8.7 mm diameter
Low lens position

9.2 mm diameter
Low lens position corrected by
lenticular design and larger size

In fitting aphakic patients (with the use of intraocular lens implants, aphakic contact lens fitting is happening much less frequently than in the past), the guidelines are similar to fitting the hyperopic eye. The larger diameters (9.7–10.5 mm) center better and are more stable than the smaller diameters. The aphakic diagnostic fitting set is:

DIAMETER	POWER	BASE CURVE RANGE (0.50-DIOPTER STEPS)
9.7 mm (lenticular)	+ 14.00 diopters	40.00 diopters (8.44 mm) to 46.00 diopters (7.34 mm)

Additional diameters of 8.7 mm (single cut) and 10.5 mm (lenticular cut) are helpful.

FITTING THE PATIENT WHO HAS BEEN WEARING HARD CONTACT LENSES

If there is significant corneal distortion as seen by keratometry and slit-lamp evaluation (Fig. 1.36), it may be necessary to discontinue all contact lens wear until there is some stabilization of the corneal topography. Otherwise a 9.2-mm lens with the base curve according to Table 1.6 is placed on the eye. This lens is modified according to the slit-lamp evaluation, with the power determined by over-refraction. Careful monitoring of the patient and the lenses will detect changes which might require that the initial lens be changed during follow-up visits.

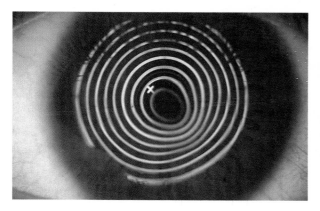

Fig. 1.36 *Corneal distortion (seen with Placido disc).*

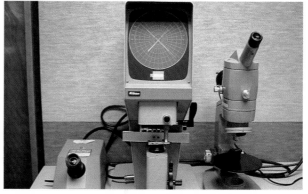

Fig. 1.37 *Instruments for analyzing and checking rigid contact lenses.*

RIGID CONTACT LENSES

It is obvious that fitting lenses is not simply taking measurements and ordering a lens. The lens must be observed on the eye at the time of the initial fitting and must be evaluated at specific intervals. When indicated, it may have to be changed. For these reasons it is not possible to examine a patient and hand him or her a contact lens prescription. The information obtained is simply the starting point for the fitting of the contact lens.

Before dispensing a contact lens it is essential to inspect the lens for correct power, base curve, and size as well as to inspect the quality of the edge design and the peripheral curves (Fig. 1.37). Quality control varies significantly from company to company and irregular quality may be the first sign of general problems in a specific company (Fig. 1.38).

FOLLOW-UP OF RIGID CONTACT LENS PATIENTS (HARD OR RGP)

After instructing the patient in the insertion, removal (Fig. 1.39), and care of the lenses, the patient usually is seen 1 to 2 weeks after the fitting, then 2–4 weeks later. The history should seek out potential problems such as comfort difficulties, poor

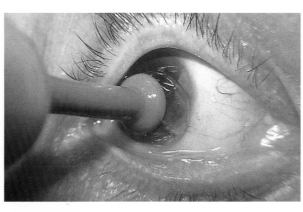

Fig. 1.39
Suction cup for removal of rigid contact lenses.

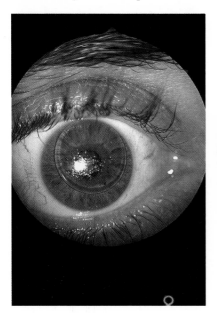

Fig. 1.38 *Greasy contact lens as received from manufacturer.*

vision, ocular redness, and spectacle blur. In addition to the above, the annual check-up should include a complete ocular examination.

It is not possible to give an accurate contact lens prescription to the patient on an initial exam. It is necessary to have adequate assessment and follow-up by completing the fitting procedure and arriving at the point when the patient is discharged until the next annual exam. The keratometer and refraction findings are the starting point. The lens may be modified at any point depending upon the reaction of the eye to the lens. Each fitter should carry out his or her own measurements and fitting and not depend upon someone else's findings.

The exam should always include visual acuity, slit-lamp evaluation with and without fluorescein, over-refraction if vision is

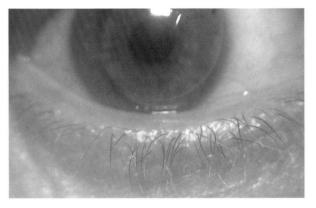

Fig. 1.40 *Fluorosilicone acrylate contact lens without fluorescein.*

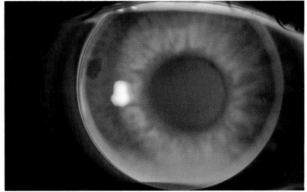

Fig. 1.41 *Fluorosilicone acrylate (Equalens) with fluorescein.*

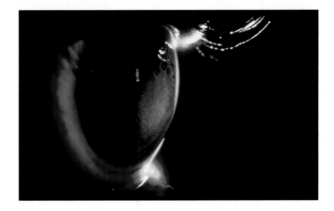

Fig. 1.42 *Corneal edema.*

RIGID CONTACT LENSES

not as expected, removal of the lenses with immediate refraction, and keratometry. This exam should be carried out later in the day. Spectacle blur and corneal distortion are not acceptable with well-fitting lenses.

Evaluation of the fluorescein pattern may be more difficult with ultraviolet (UV) absorbing materials (Fig. 1.40), especially with the newer aspheric designs which are fit flatter than the standard lenses that have been discussed in this chapter (Fig. 1.41). The fit of the aspheric lenses are monitored by observation of the fluorescein pattern, with a goal of achieving minimal apical bearing.

COMPLICATIONS OF RIGID LENS FITTING

The cornea is kept in a deturgesced state by a metabolically driven pump that requires oxygen. Under anoxic conditions, this pump no longer functions effectively, and corneal swelling ensues. The signs of corneal anoxia include conjunctival injection and central corneal edema (Fig. 1.42), which is best seen with the slit-lamp beam that is set for specular illumination (Fig. 1.43). The symptoms of this edema include halos around point light sources and spectacle blur (blurred vision with glasses upon removing the contact lenses). Treatment includes diameter re-

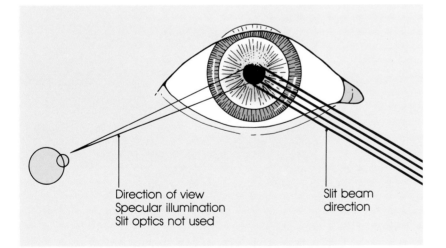

Fig. 1.43 *Specular illumination to view corneal edema.*

duction, peripheral curve blending (Fig. 1.44), and fenestration holes (Fig. 1.45) drilled in the contact lens. This edema is rare with gas-permeable lenses.

Corneal epithelial irregularities and staining (Fig. 1.46) with fluorescein may occur and will require changing the size or base curve of the lens. If uncorrected, corneal scarring may occur (Fig. 1.47). Three and nine o'clock staining may be caused by corneal drying (Fig. 1.48). Treatment consists of diameter al-

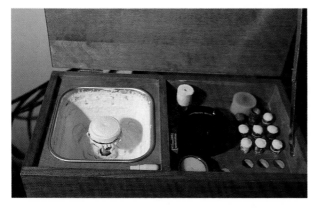

Fig. 1.44 *Kit for modifying rigid lenses in the office.*

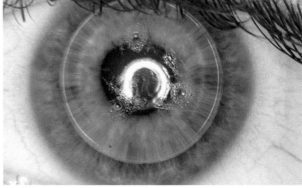

Fig. 1.45 *Fenestrated rigid contact lens, with holes plugged with debris.*

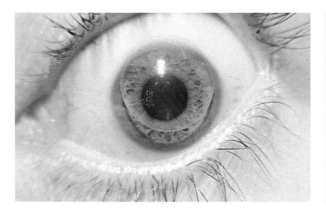

Fig. 1.46 *Contact lens keratopathy.*

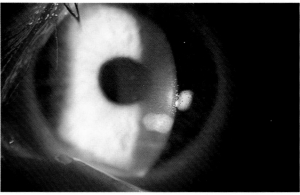

Fig. 1.47 *Scarring of cornea.*

teration, artificial tears and wetting agents, and peripheral and intermediate curve blending. It may be necessary to change to a different RGP material.

Apical dot staining appears with early corneal edema (Fig. 1.46). Poor lens quality, inadvertent touching the cornea upon insertion or removal, or foreign bodies trapped under the contact lens may cause linear or solid staining of the cornea (Fig. 1.49).

Poorly centering lenses and intolerance of solutions (Figs. 1.50 and 1.51) may be responsible for uncomfortable lenses. Corneal

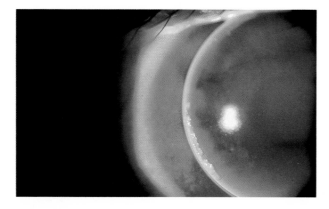

Fig. 1.48 *Three and nine o'clock staining.*

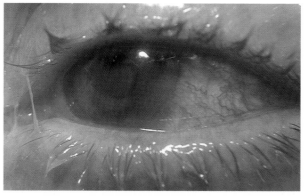

Fig. 1.49 *Corneal staining from finger abrasion.*

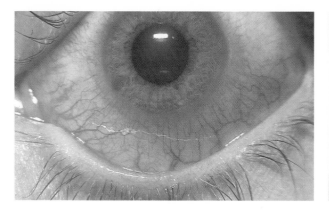

Fig. 1.50 *Thimerosal sensitivity.*

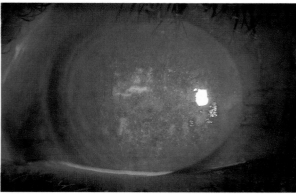

Fig. 1.51 *Keratopathy from solution reaction.*

staining may occur with flat or steep lenses or with overwearing (Fig. 1.52). Lenses that are too small may cause the patient to experience flare and to see the edge of the lenses. Flexure of the lens (bending) may cause unstable vision. Poor manufacturing techniques and poor edge design are responsible for uncomfortable lenses.

Vascularization of the cornea may be produced by either chronic anoxia or contact-lens-induced irritation, showing up in the form of a circumlimbal pannus (Fig. 1.53) with a predilection for vessels to invade the peripheral cornea superiorly (Fig. 1.54). This may progress to infiltration of the pannus toward the central cornea. After removing the lens, ghost vessels or corneal scarring may remain. As with all contact lenses, especially with poor hygiene and poor care, serious corneal infections may occur (Fig. 1.55).

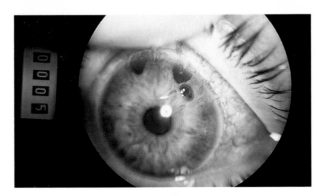

Fig. 1.52 *Keratopathy from overwearing of contact lens.*

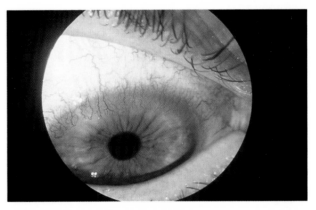

Fig. 1.53 *Corneal pannus.*

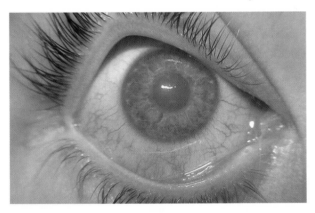

Fig. 1.54 *Intracorneal hemorrhage from vascularization of cornea.*

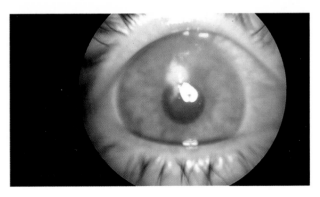

Fig. 1.55 *Infectious corneal ulcer.*

RIGID CONTACT LENSES

Although they may occur much less frequently than with soft lenses, deposits may form on the surface of rigid lenses (Fig. 1.56). The same applies to giant papillary conjunctivitis (GPC) (Fig. 1.57).

All of the above complications were more common with hard PMMA lenses than with gas-permeable lenses.

SUMMARY

Fitting contact lenses is an art that may be initiated by following some guidelines and being aware of the properties and limitations of lenses. In order to achieve greater success and safety for patients, the fitter must be constantly alert and continually evaluate the fit of the lenses.

ACKNOWLEDGMENTS

The authors would like to thank Sue Mullett and Ruth Clemens of Canton Ophthalmology Associates, Inc., for their assistance in the preparation of Chapters 1 and 6.

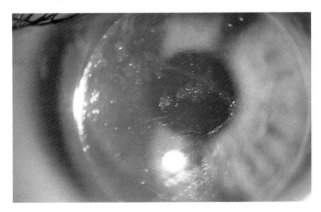

Fig. 1.56 *Deposits on rigid gas-permeable contact lens.*

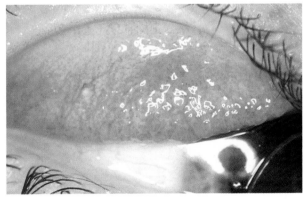

Fig. 1.57 *Giant papillary conjunctivitis (GPC).*

REFERENCES

1. Rosenthal, Perry. Quoted in *Opthalmology Times* issue of 4/1/86.

2. Girard, L. J., Sampson, W. J., and Soper, J. W. *Corneal Contact Lenses*, Mosby, St. Louis, 1966.

3. Franklin, J. B. CAB lenses in aphakia. In: Emery, J. (Ed.) *Current Controversies in Cataract Surgery*, Mosby, St. Louis, pp. 47–48, 1978.

4. Barr, J. T., and Schoessler, J. P. Corneal endothelial response to rigid contact lenses. *Am. J. Optom. Physiol. Opt.*, 57(5):267, 1980.

5. Miller, D., and Weiss, J. N. Corneal endothelium. *Int. Ophthalmol. Clin.*, 21:2, 1981.

6. Allensmith, M., et al. Giant papillary conjunctivitis in contact lens wearers. *Am. J. Ophthalmol.*, 83:697, 1977.

7. Donshik, Peter C. Personal communication, 1986.

8. Norman, Craig V., and Caroline, Patrick J. A Basic Guide to Contact Lens Fitting. Personal course hand-out material.

2
SOFT CONTACT LENSES

MICHAEL A. LEMP, M.D.
DIANN E. PINNER-RYAN, C.O.T.

In an effort to meet the visual needs of the growing contact lens population, we now have (a) soft lenses for myopia, hyperopia, astigmatism, presbyopia, and aphakia, (b) cosmetic tints to change eye color, and (c) cosmesis reclamation. In this chapter we shall review the prefitting, fitting, and follow-up care of these widely used lenses (Fig. 2.1).

INDICATIONS

Soft contact lenses are indicated for motivated patients who (a) desire soft lenses, (b) cannot tolerate or do not want rigid lenses, (c) may desire intermittent or extended wear, and (d) have refractive errors.

Although spherical lenses correct a minimal amount of astigmatism, toric lenses are available, as are bifocal and multifocal lenses (see Chapters 6 and 7).

CONTRAINDICATIONS

Soft lenses are contraindicated if good vision or comfort are not obtainable, in patients with poor hygiene and in patients with topical or systemic disease conditions as mentioned below.

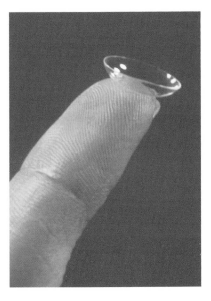

Fig. 2.1 *Soft lens.*

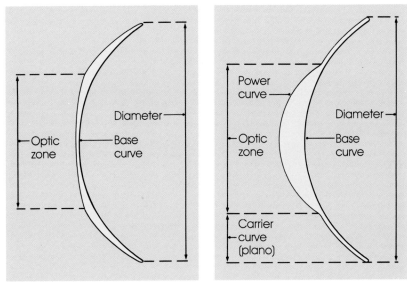

Fig. 2.2 *Minus soft lens profile.*

Fig. 2.3 *Aphakic soft lens profile.*

SOFT CONTACT LENSES

MATERIALS AND MARKET

Soft lenses are made of a variety of copolymers ranging in water content from 35% to 79%. Each lens contains a polymer combination with unique qualities. The polymers are arranged in varying densities and structures. This allows each lens to have different properties of water content, oxygen transmissibility, surface wetability, and durability. Designs vary in curvature (relating to overall diameter), thickness (relating to water content), optical zone (relating to overall diameter), and edge design. There is an increasing number of different brand names on the market today. Of these, some are of the same polymeric material but cut in different designs (Figs. 2.2 and 2.3). The neophyte in lens fitting is faced with the difficult task of learning about the myriad of brands and designs in the marketplace today. We believe that any office can meet the fitting needs of 90% of the population by choosing two soft lens companies that have different designs and materials. Examples of this would be: Bausch & Lomb and Cooper Vision; Hydrocurve and Bausch & Lomb; Ciba and Cooper Vision; Wesley–Jessen and American Hydron.

METHODS OF MANUFACTURE

There are three methods of manufacturing soft lenses: spin casting, cast molding, and lathe cutting. Spin casting is the technique used by Bausch & Lomb for its Soflens. A combination of spin casting the front surface and lathe cutting the back surface is used for the Bausch & Lomb Optima lens. Cast molding is the method used for the American Optical lens, now owned by Ciba. Most other lenses are lathe cut in a dehydrated state and, when finished, rehydrated (Fig. 2.4).

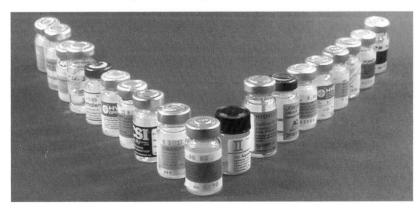

Fig. 2.4 *Assortment of soft lenses.*

CLASSIFICATIONS

Soft lenses can be divided into two classifications: daily wear and extended wear. These two classifications can be further divided into two categories based on water content and thickness. A high-water-content lens has to be cut thick, to prevent disintegration, but a low-water-content lens can be cut either thick (with less oxygen transmission) or thin (with more oxygen transmission). Each lens has a personality of its own. This personality is defined by the problem situation it will solve.

DAILY WEAR

The water content of a daily-wear contact lens ranges from 35% to 50%. Of the many designs, all can be categorized as either thick or thin or can be divided in reference to their size: small, medium, or large.

Thick lenses mask more astigmatism within limits. The thicker the lens, the more rigidity it possesses, and therefore it neutralizes a larger amount of corneal astigmatism. This type of lens is also easier for the patient to handle.

The trade-off for using a thicker lens for masking astigmatism and better vision is possible corneal molding, particularly in minus powers higher than -4.00. Corneal molding is defined as a rapid unexplained increase in myopia after soft lens fitting and will be explained more fully at the end of the chapter, in the section on follow-up problem solving. Examples of this are Aquaflex Standard, AO Standard, Softcon DW, and American Hydron.

The second category of the daily-wear lenses is the thin (lower water content) lens. This type of lens is referred to as a *membrane lens* and has the advantageous quality of "draping" over the cornea. The membrane lenses have thin edges for comfort and good centration. This type of lens also requires less movement because oxygen is more efficiently delivered as a result of the thinness of the lens. Well-known lenses in this category are: Bausch & Lomb Ultrathin series, Syntex CSI T, Hydron Zero-4, Cooper Vision Permathin series, and Cibathin series. The disadvantage of a thin lens is difficulty in handling.

The third category of daily-wear lenses is the large-diameter soft lens. This type of lens ranges in diameter from 15.0 to 16.0 mm. Its primary purpose is problem-solving for large corneal diameters, more complete corneal coverage, tight lids, or wide palpebral fissure spaces. Better stability and comfort are achieved when a larger portion of the lens is tucked up under the upper lid. The disadvantage of the large diameter is difficulty in insertion if the palpebral fissure space is not wide enough; large-diameter lenses are also disadvantageous for people with porched brows, which prevent separating the lids far enough apart for insertion. One of the few large-diameter designs is manufactured by Hydrocurve.

The fourth category of daily-wear lenses is the small–medium-diameter soft lens. We define the range of this diameter to be 12.5–14.5 mm. The majority of soft lenses are within this range and will suit the needs of most fittings.

EXTENDED-WEAR SOFT LENSES (EWSL)

Soft lenses qualify as extended-wear lenses by providing sufficient oxygen to sustain corneal metabolism overnight. FDA studies were completed for each EWSL on the market today. It is prudent to remember, however, that the patients in these studies did well under the perfect and stringent guidelines of many and frequent follow-up visits as prescribed by strict protocol. Recently, concern has arisen over adverse pathologic findings in the EWSL wearers.

EWSLs permit sufficient oxygen transmissibility to provide for minimal corneal respiratory needs either by their (a) high water content or (b) thinness (membrane lens). The exception is when a lens is a combination of both with a little more water content and a little less thickness than daily-wear soft lenses.

ADVANTAGES/DISADVANTAGES

1. A high-water-content lens (70% and above) gives excellent transmission of oxygen but is more fragile, resulting in a higher incidence of lens damage and more frequent wear-out.
2. A thin-membrane lens (low in water content, 30–40%) facilitates oxygen transmission by thinness but is harder for the patient to handle for insertion in the low powers (below −2.00) because of its "Saran Wrap-like" quality. Damage often occurs when the lens folds and sticks to itself. Extended-wear powers in the thin lenses usually end at −6.00 or −7.00.
3. A medium-water-content lens (55–60%) is easier for the patient to handle but gives less oxygen transmission when fit in the higher powers.

SOFT CONTACT LENSES

The characteristics of examples of some of the different EWSL designs mentioned above are summarized in Table 2.1.

PREFITTING EVALUATION

If a thorough and complete prefitting examination of the patient is done before lens trial, it will invariably save you and the patient multiple follow-up visits beyond the routine requirement. The importance of this part of the fitting process cannot be stressed enough. Experience has taught us all that the 15 min saved on initial exam might come back to haunt us months afterwards and (three sets of lenses later) when we are still struggling to fit the "mysteriously difficult" patients.

HISTORY—OPHTHALMIC

A careful history of current ocular diagnosis and therapy as well as a past history of ocular injury, surgery, amblyopia therapy, infection, or episodic symptoms of itching, burning, or tearing, either seasonal or chronic, should be obtained from the patient. List any over-the-counter eye preparations used by the patient. Patients should be made aware that most of these preparations cannot be used while wearing soft lenses.

TABLE 2.1
EXAMPLES OF EXTENDED WEAR SOFT LENS CHARACTERISTICS (MINUS)

High Water Content		Thin (Low Water Content)		Combination Medium Water	
Permalens	71% water (CT 0.23)	Bausch & Lomb 03,04	38% water (0.035 CT)	Softmate II	55% water (CT 0.05)
Bausch & Lomb 70	70% water (CT 0.14)	CSI T	38.5% water (0.035 CT)	Softcon EW	55% water (CT 0.06)
		Permaflex Thin	43% water (0.035 CT)		
		Hydron Zero-4	36% water (0.04 CT)		

HISTORY—SYSTEMIC

The patient's medical history can reveal a good deal of information that may affect the success or lack of success in soft lens wear.

Patients with chronic allergies to household elements or seasonal allergies will have more difficulty and will probably have to discontinue use of soft lenses during times of ocular symptoms.

It is important to note specific systemic disorders and medications associated with their therapy. For example, patients with hypertension and/or heart disease may be treated with various medications containing diuretics or beta blockers. These medications significantly decrease body hydration and possibly decrease tear production. Patients with depressive disorders may be taking tricyclic antidepressants. These medications may cause a dry eye syndrome and create a poor ocular surface for soft contact lenses. Diabetic patients may have varying degrees of corneal anesthesia. Contact lenses are generally contraindicated in this clinical situation, since patients are more prone to developing neurotropic keratitis and secondary infections. Patients with rheumatoid arthritis and related collagen vascular disorders may have a Sjogren's syndrome with keratoconjunctivitis sicca and associated tear film abnormalities. Patients with irritable bowel syndrome (spastic colon) may be using an anticholinergic (e.g., Pro-Banthine), which decreases tear production. Drug therapy for acne (i.e., Acutane) may cause reduced tear production. Soft lenses should be discontinued during the course of treatment. Alcohol abuse may contraindicate the use of soft lenses. Changes in the patient's body hydration due to frequent diuresis will adversely affect the soft lens hydration. Remember, the relative hydration of a soft lens must be maintained by adequate tear production. Decreased hydration of a soft lens will result in the lens steepening while being worn.

EXTRAOCULAR OBSERVATIONS

The presence of small, spiderlike telangiectatic vessels in the skin over the cheeks and over the bridge of the nose may indicate an underlying dermatological condition known as *acne rosacea*, which is associated with chronic blepharitis. Both a penlight and slit-lamp examination of the eyelid skin, eyelashes, and lid margins can quickly detect conditions that may adversely affect contact lens wear, including: the presence of misdirected lashes;

the presence of crusting and debris surrounding the individual cilia (collarettes) (Fig. 2.5); irregularities of the lid margin; and foamy discharge in the medial or lateral canthi, indicating an angular blepharitis or dilated telangiectatic vessels in the eyelid skin or surrounding the eyelashes, which may also indicate blepharitis. Chronic blepharitis, tear film abnormalities, meibomian gland dysfunction with abnormal fatty acid composition of the lipid component of the tear film, and secondary keratoconjunctivitis sicca with punctate keratopathy may all be secondary to rosacea blepharitis (Fig. 2.6). The presence of rhinophyma due to sebaceous gland abnormalities in the skin of the nose may also indicate the presence of rosacea and coexisting blepharitis.

STRUCTURAL VARIATIONS THAT AFFECT SOFT LENS FITTING

The challenge of soft lens fitting is continually new with the variables in each patient. Over the years, it has become apparent that certain quantifiable measurements in conjunction with subtle (nonmeasurable) variations in orbital and facial structure have to be taken into consideration when choosing the most effective soft lens. Listed below are prefitting measurements of which the first three are quantifiable and the last four are simple observations to be noted on the chart only if present.

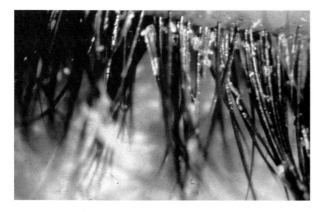

Fig. 2.5 *Lashes with collarettes.*

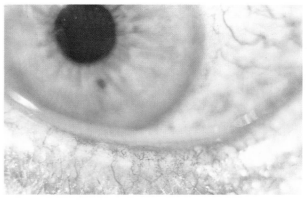

Fig. 2.6 *Rosacea blepharitis.*

SOFT CONTACT LENSES

1. Palpebral fissure space—in millimeters
2. Corneal diameter—in millimeters
3. Pupil size—in millimeters
4. Globe shape—estimated to be long or short
5. Lids—tight or lax, heavy or post-blepharoplasty
6. Orbital bone structure—deep-set, porched brows, widely spaced eyes (telecanthus)
7. Prominence of globe—proptotic or recessed

1. *Palpebral fissure space:* Vertical measurement of the opening between the upper and lower lids will help determine the appropriate size of a soft lens (Fig. 2.7). If the palpebral fissure space measurement is small, the patient may not be able to open the lids far enough apart to insert a medium- or large-diameter lens. A smaller soft lens (i.e., 13.0 or 13.5 mm) will help alleviate this problem. Some examples of small-diameter lenses are: Hydron Mini, Flexlens, Omegasoft, and Aquaflex standard minus. A patient with an abnormally large palpebral fissure space (Fig. 2.8) will need a larger lens to tuck up under the upper lid for stability. Examples are Hydrocurve 15–16-mm lens or CSI 14.8-mm lens.

A lens will orient with the apical center of the cornea but will be pulled toward the widest portion of the palpebral fissure space with the blink. Therefore, if the widest point of the palpebral fissure is not at the same point directly above the corneal apex, the lens will be pulled off center toward the widest point of the palpebral fissure space, usually temporally. When the lens

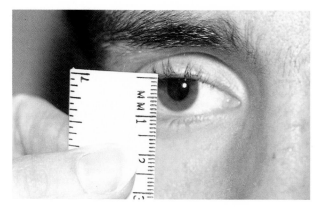

Fig. 2.7 *Measuring vertical palpebral fissure space.*

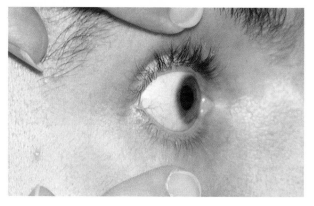

Fig. 2.8 *View of corneal profile.*

is large enough, the pupil will remain within the optical zone (Fig. 2.9).

2. *Corneal diameter:* Corneal diameters may range from 10.0 to 13.0 mm. A soft lens with a small diameter (i.e., 13.0–13.5 mm) placed on a large cornea (i.e., 13.0 mm) will irritate the limbus, causing conjunctival injection and discomfort. Complete corneal coverage should be achieved.

3. *Pupil size:* Pupils should be measured in low light in millimeters, and documentation should be made of any abnormalities. A high myope with large pupils will be more comfortable with a larger optical zone, particularly in low light conditions when the pupils are dilated (e.g., driving at night). Pupillary abnormalities may influence the choice of lens design. Patients with updrawn pupils will do better with a larger optical zone in a soft lens (Fig. 2.10).

4. *Globe shape:* A gross estimate of the globe shape is necessary for soft lens fitting. The hyperoptic patient with average or steep keratometric measurements will have to be fit with a much flatter base curve than suspected by K-readings. If the short focal length is not due to a flat cornea, it is usually due to a short globe. The short globe is associated with a much flatter sclera, upon which the periphery of the soft lens will sit. Therefore, a flatter lens may be needed than is indicated by the K-readings. Conversely, the myopic patient with average or flat K-values will usually have a long globe, causing a drastic drop off at the sclera.

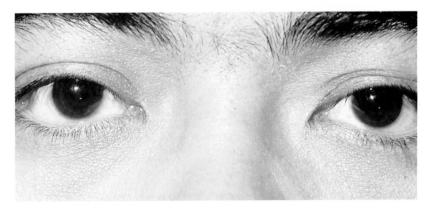

Fig. 2.9 *Center of cornea not aligned with widest portion of palpebral fissure space.*

The best way to assess this is to fully open both lids with your fingers and look at the relationships in profile (Figs. 2.11 and 2.12). This will help to decide which trial lens to first use.

5. *Lids:* An assessment of lid tightness, laxity, and effective closure should be made in the prefitting examination. Grasping the upper lid between thumb and forefinger and gently pulling outward will give the fitter an estimation of lid tension over the globe. Tight lids will pull a contact lens upward. Heavy or fatty upper lids will displace a lens downward. Post-blepharoplasty lid tightness or incomplete lid closure with blink should be noted. To maintain full hydration, the lid must distribute the tear film completely.

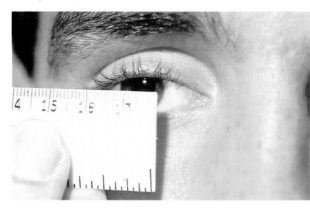

Fig. 2.10 *Horizontal measurement of corneal diameter.*

Fig. 2.11 *Parting lids to look at corneal profile.*

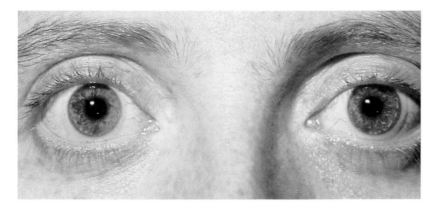

Fig. 2.12 *Large palpebral fissure spaces.*

6. *Orbital bone structure:* Variations in orbital and facial bone structure should be considered. Patients with deep-set eyes, small palpebral fissure spaces, and small fornices (Fig. 2.13) may have difficulty with lens insertion and removal as do patients with prominent superior orbital rims (porched brows) (Fig. 2.14).

7. *Prominence of globe:* Prominent or proptotic eyes have to be considered with both hard and soft lens fittings. (Fig. 2.15). Check for complete lid closure. The upper eyelid must extend both outward and over a prominent globe (Fig. 2.16); therefore, greater lid excursion may require the use of a larger size soft lens with thin edges as in the Bausch & Lomb U4 14.5 mm, CSI 14.8 mm, and Hydrocurve II 15.5 mm.

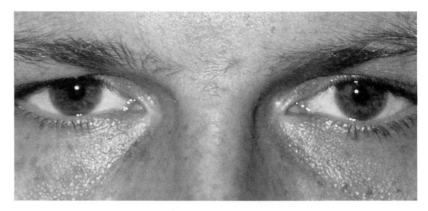

Fig. 2.13 *Patient with small palpebral fissure spaces.*

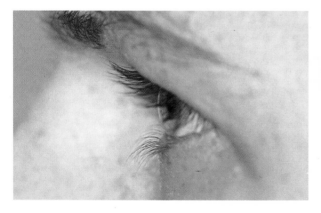

Fig. 2.14 *Prominent superior orbital rims (porched brows).*

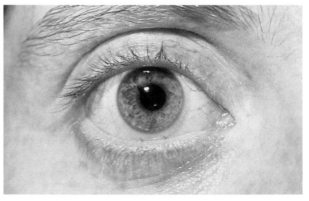

Fig. 2.15 *Prominent or proptotic eyes.*

SOFT CONTACT LENSES

SLIT-LAMP OBSERVATIONS

The bulbar conjunctiva is examined for evidence of hyperemia. Neovascularization of the cornea is exacerbated by soft contact lens wear; evidence of this, particularly by the patient who has formerly worn lenses (Fig. 2.17), should be measured and noted. The presence of pingueculae or pterygia generally contraindicates the wear of soft lenses (Fig. 2.18). This should be explained to the patient. The tarsal conjunctiva of the upper and lower eyelids should be inspected for the presence of giant papillary conjunctivitis (GPC) (Fig. 2.19).

A quick look at the marginal tear strip or the lacrimal lake will give a gross evaluation of the adequacy of tears. An important observation about the tears is the presence of mucus, debris, and oil. Soft contact lenses attract mucus, debris, and

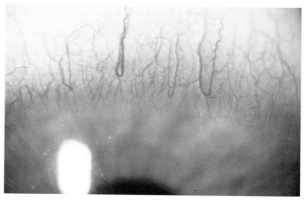

Fig. 2.16 *Profile of prominent or proptotic eyes.*

Fig. 2.17 *Neovascularization of superior cornea.*

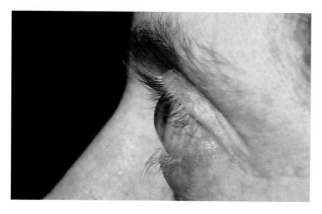

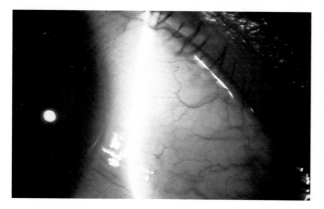

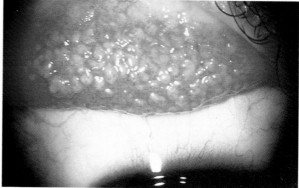

Fig. 2.18 *Pingueculae.*

Fig. 2.19 *Everted lid with giant papillary conjunctivitis.*

oil like a magnet, causing film buildup on the front surface of the lens. The patient will experience minimum to moderate success with visual acuity in the lenses and must be counseled for shorter wear-time with more frequent enzymatic cleaning.

The tear break-up time (TBUT) is also an important indicator of overall tear quality. TBUT refers to the time it takes for the appearance of dark, nonfluorescent dots in the tear film after instilling fluorescein and keeping the eyelids open. A TBUT of less than 8 sec should be noted as an indicator for comfort problems that might be encountered during the fitting process. This alone does not contraindicate soft lens fitting; however, in conjunction with low Schirmer test and/or mucus and debris in the tear film, the overall success rate is diminished substantially.

The cornea should be examined for any positive or negative fluorescein staining. If staining is found, the pathogenesis must be established before continuing with routine soft lens fitting.

All existing lid, corneal, conjunctival, iris, pupil, and lens defects should be noted for future reference in follow-up. The presence of a filtering bleb contraindicates the fitting of a soft lens because the lens may predispose the patient to severe intraocular infection.

SCHIRMER TEST

A Schirmer test should be performed prior to all contact lens fittings (Fig. 2.20). This documentation can save the fitter many hours of follow-up time. A Schirmer test is a gross estimation of tear production at best, but truly dry eyes (less than 8 mm of

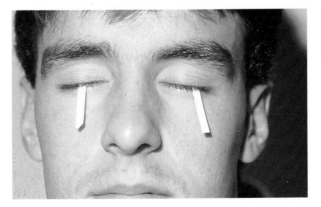

Fig. 2.20 *Schirmer strip test being performed.*

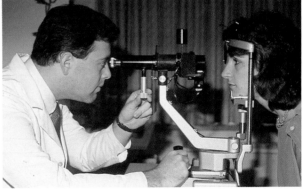

Fig. 2.21 *Ophthalmometer measurements being taken.*

wetting) will invariably have difficulty with soft lens wear. As mentioned before, dryness can be pathogenic or drug induced, and the relative hydration of a soft lens must be maintained by adequate tear production. With the presence of a low Schirmer test, the lower-water-content lens will achieve the best results. An example of one such lens is the Syntex SCI lens.

KERATOMETER/OPHTHALMOMETER MEASUREMENTS

Careful recording of the corneal curvature with a keratometer or ophthalmometer should be done on the initial exam before applanation or indentation tonography is performed (Fig. 2.21). Applanation or indentation will distort the corneal mires, giving a false flattening and/or warping appearance. The keratometer/ophthalmometer measurements should be taken before doing a refraction, to differentiate refractive astigmatism from the measured corneal astigmatism and, more importantly, to reveal lenticular astigmatism. This will play an important role in the choice between fitting a spherical soft lens and having to fit an astigmatic soft lens to correct the lenticular astigmatism.

FITTING TECHNIQUE

The essential ingredient of soft lens fitting is diagnostic trial lenses (Fig. 2.22). A complete range of curvatures and a limited range of powers (both from the same manufacturer) are needed

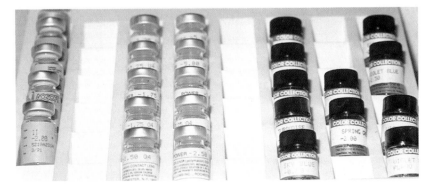

Fig. 2.22 *Diagnostic trial lenses.*

to accomplish the initial fitting and later to solve subtle and often obscure problems in follow-up exams. Unlike hard lenses, soft lenses are manufactured in specific parameters of curvature, power range and diameter.

INITIAL LENS CHOICE

Based on the pre-exam and discussion with the patient, the choice between daily wear and extended wear has to be made. Based on structural physiologic variations of the patient's eyes, the fitter will choose the type of lens that will best meet the limitations present.

The base curves offered by any manufacturer can easily be broken down into three categories: flat, medium, and steep. Because the companies wish to capture the majority of fits in the average population, they have already designed and marketed their lenses to meet the range.

The first fitting step is to categorize the patient's keratometer/ophthalmometer measurements into one of the three fits: *flat, medium,* or *steep.*

A rule of thumb for K-reading in diopters is:

FLAT	MEDIUM	STEEP	
41.00–42.75	43.00–44.75	45.00–46.75	and above

An example of this initial lens selection is as follows:

CIBA—13.8-MM DIAMETER			**HYDRON ZERO-6—14.0-MM DIAMETER**		
FLAT	MEDIUM	STEEP	FLAT	MEDIUM	STEEP
BC 8.9	BC 8.6	BC 8.3	BC 9.0	BC 8.7	BC 8.4

Some companies will offer only two selections from which to choose a proper fit. In that case, consult with the marketing representatives and ask specifically which lens best fits the flat, medium, and steep range of curvature. An example of this is as follows:

COOPER PERMAFLEX—14.4-MM DIAMETER		**BAUSCH & LOMB OPTIMA**	
FLAT AND MEDIUM	STEEP	FLAT & MEDIUM	STEEP
8.9 BC	8.7	Sag I	Sag II

The Bausch & Lomb spin-cast lens (U3, U4, O3, O4) does not follow any of the above rules. The base curvature of a spin-cast lens will change as the power changes upward or downward. It is essential that the Bausch & Lomb spin-cast lens be trial-fit within 0.75 diopters of the needed power. The most utilized fits of the Bausch & Lomb spin-cast lenses are the U3 and U4 series and the O3–O4 series. The U3 and O3 series is 13.5 mm in diameter and will generally fit the flatter cornea, whereas the U4 and O4 series is 14.5 mm in diameter and will generally fit the medium-to-steep cornea.

Again, remember, the K readings can be very deceiving. The curvature readings are of the central 5 mm of the cornea. The soft lens rests outside the limbus, and this curvature is quite different. As mentioned previously, parting the lids and observing the contour of the sclera as well as the contour of the cornea will give you an estimate of the need for a flat, medium, or steep lens (Fig. 2.23).

EVALUATION OF FIT *IN SITU*:

After the initial lens has been placed on the eye, the patient should sit for 20–45 min to allow the lens to equilibrate and to allow the patient to cease initial reflex tearing. The higher the water content in the lens, the longer the lens should be allowed to equilibrate (for aphakic EWSLs, a few hours of equilibration are needed before evaluation can be accurately performed). The next step is to evaluate the movement and centration of the lens on the eye.

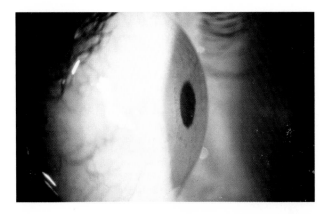

Fig. 2.23 *Profile of corneal/scleral relationship.*

GOOD FIT OBSERVATIONS

1. Almost perfect centration when the eye is in straight normal gaze and when the lids are held apart (Fig. 2.24).
2. The lens should move with each blink: 0.5–1 mm of movement with the membrane lenses; 1–2 mm of movement with the standard thickness lenses. In upgaze, the movement should double.
3. The lens should rapidly return to centration after a shift in gaze.
4. The entire cornea should be covered by the lens, and the edge of the lens should not ride beyond the limbus and into the cornea with normal blink.

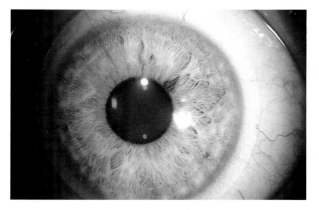

Fig. 2.24 *Well-centered lens in straight gaze.*

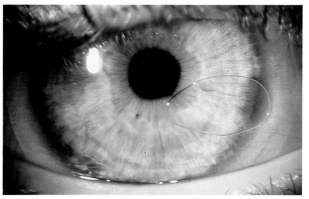

Fig. 2.25 *Bubble trapped under lens—too steep fit.*

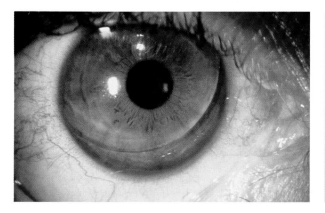

Fig. 2.26 *Lens decentered superiorly—too flat fit.*

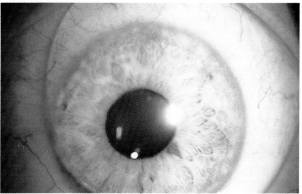

Fig. 2.27 *Lens with edge stand-off—extremely flat fit.*

POOR FIT—TOO STEEP
1. Bubbles seen trapped under lens (Fig. 2.25), or
2. Less than 0.5-mm movement with blink; conjunctival folds are shoved, but lens does not "slide" freely. Same amount of movement or lack of movement in upgaze.
3. Redness of conjunctiva at border of lens or scleral indentation after removal of lens.
4. Patient will report that vision is briefly clear after blink but then fades.

POOR FIT—TOO LOOSE
1. Excessive movement with each "normal" blink. There is a lag time (1–2 sec) before lens returns to centration.
2. Lower edge is pulled up beyond limbus in primary gaze. (Fig. 2.26).
3. Edge stand off (Fig. 2.27).
4. The patient will report that acuity is poor after each blink and then comes in after 1–2 sec.

OVER-REFRACTION
After a properly fit lens is determined, the fitter can proceed with the over-refraction. The first step is plusing and minusing with hand-held spherical lenses. If the expected optimum vision is not achieved with spherical over-refraction, the fitter should use a retinoscope to check for residual astigmatism. At this point, it is important to *show* the patient what can and cannot be achieved with spherical soft lens correction (Fig. 2.28) and discuss the alternatives of astigmatic soft lens fitting and hard lens fitting. Different patients will accept varying degrees of vision;

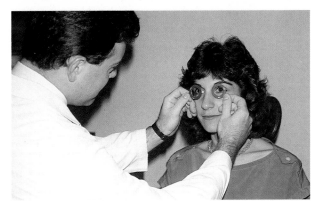

Fig. 2.28 *Demonstrating vision potential to patient with over-refraction.*

it is therefore important for the fitter to discuss possibilities, as well as limitations, before the initial order is placed. Having the patient participate and understand your fitting decisions at this point will save frustration and false expectations in the follow-up visits to come.

FOLLOW-UP PROBLEM SOLVING

The initial selecting and trial fitting of a soft lens is the first hurdle in successful lens fitting. Often, the real challenge comes with the second and third follow-up visits. Problem solving for the formerly successful lens wearer, frequently seen after an emergency room visit, can be equally as challenging. Listening to the patient's symptoms and tediously reviewing what the patient does and doesn't do with his/her lenses will play a key role in solving the mysteries that can be related to objective findings.

The following are some of the common problems seen with lens fittings and follow-up:

1. *Staining:* Corneal staining after lens wear can be caused by: anoxia (Fig. 2.29) due to structurally damaged lens (spoilage from age and/or deposits); tight lens; nicked lens; trapped debris; chemical keratitis from solutions; poor insertion and removal technique (mechanically inflicted staining) (Fig. 2.30); or corneal exposure (incomplete corneal coverage or incomplete blinking).

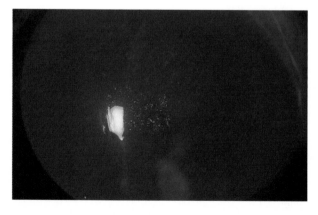

Fig. 2.29 *Corneal staining after soft lens wear.*

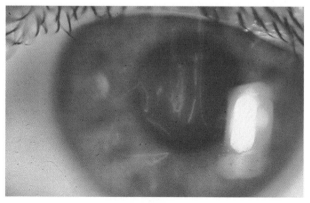

Fig. 2.30 *Mechanically inflicted corneal staining.*

SOFT CONTACT LENSES

2. *Red burning eyes:* Causes include: tight lens; solution sensitivities; improper rinsing of lens before insertion; dry eyes; or structurally damaged lenses (spoilage from age or deposits) (Figs. 2.31 and 2.32).

3. *Constant lens awareness:* Causes include: loose lens fit with too much movement; defective or nicked lens edge; lens too small or too thick; inverted lens.

4. *Unexplained increase in myopia:* Higher-than-expected increases of myopia in a patient fit within the last few months should be investigated. After systemic or cataract changes have been ruled out, the usual cause is from a thick lens or a tight lens causing corneal molding. Confirmation of this is a steepening of K-readings or increase in corneal astigmatism. This situation is relieved by simply refitting with a flatter, thinner, or higher-water-content lens. The refractive error should return to original value within 1 or 2 weeks of lens discontinuation.

5. *Lens spoilage or wear-out:* It is important to ascertain the age of the soft lenses being worn by the patient. All lenses have a life span. With good care, daily-wear lenses can be expected to last for 1 year or more. This will vary, depending on care and handling and the patient's individual tear physiology. You should be reasonably suspicious of a daily-wear lens that is older than 1 year. The life span of extended-wear lenses will range from 2 months to 1 year, depending upon the care, handling, tear physiology, polymer, and water content of the lens. Higher-water-content lenses deteriorate faster. It is not uncommon for extended-wear patients to have to renew their lenses every 3–

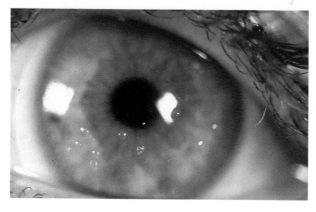

Fig. 2.31 *Soft lens deposits.*

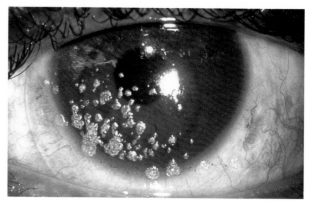

Fig. 2.32 *Severe soft lens deposits.*

SOFT CONTACT LENSES

2.21

6 months. For both daily-wear and extended-wear lenses, "lens wear-out" is not easily viewed with the slit lamp (Fig. 2.33). The lens must be removed and rinsed in the palm of the hand to appreciate a rubbery-like dragging feeling of the plastic. This is not the same as easily visualized deposits, which are easily seen in the slit lamp. Patients will commonly complain of decreased wear time; they also will complain that their lenses move more with shifting gaze, that the upper lid feels a dragging sensation over the lens, and that sometimes redness and mucous secretions occur. Most importantly, the patient remembers that the lens did not feel like this in the beginning.

REFERENCES

1. Lemp, M. A., Gold, J. B., and Pinner, D. E. Prefitting evaluation of contact lens patients. In: Stenson, S. M. (Ed.), *Contact Lenses, A Guide to Selection, Fitting and Management of Complications*, Chapter 1, Appleton & Lange, Norwalk, Connecticut, 1987.

2. Lemp, M. A., and Hamill, J. Factors affecting tear film breakup in normals. *Arch. Ophthalmol.*, 89:103–105, 1973.

3. Weissman, B. A. *Contact Lens Primer—A Manual*, Lea & Febiger, Philadelphia, 1984.

4. Tyler, Thompson, *Tyler's Quarterly*, Soft Contact Lens Parameter Guide, June 1987, Little Rock, Arkansas.

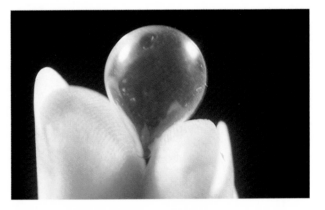

Fig. 2.33 *Structurally damaged or aged soft lens.*

3
DISPOSABLE CONTACT LENSES

SHELDON WECHSLER, M.S., O.D., F.A.A.O.

The concept of disposable contact lenses was developed in an effort to overcome the difficulties associated with extended-wear lenses. Because of problems such as corneal ulcers and Acanthamoeba keratitis, some doctors have become reluctant to prescribe lenses for extended wear. The problems have arisen, in large part, because of deposit buildup, poor patient compliance, and poor patient hygiene. The result has been that many practitioners have chosen alternate forms of vision correction, even though extended wear offers important advantages.

A recent development that addresses these problems is a lens designed to be worn continuously for a prescribed period (e.g., 1 or 2 weeks) and then replaced rather than cleaned. Based on the concepts of disposability and continuous replacement, the Acuvue lens used in conjunction with the Disposalens System was developed. This chapter will describe the disposable-lens system.

The Acuvue lens is a 58%-water-content hydrogel lens. The lens is available in the following parameters:

BASE CURVE	DIAMETER	CENTER THICKNESS (− 3.00 DIOPTERS)
8.80 mm	14.0 mm	0.07 mm

POWER (0.25-DIOPTER INCREMENTS)
− 0.50 to − 6.00 diopters

The oxygen permeability (D_k) of the Acuvue lens material is 28×10^{-11} (cm^2/sec)(ml O$_2$/mm Hg).

The lens is molded using a unique "stabilized soft molding" process. In all present manufacturing methods the hydrogel lenses are produced in the hard state and then hydrated. The soft molding process keeps the lens in the soft state during manufacture, which reduces the magnitude of parameter changes that normally occur during hydration.

The lens and the disposable system are indicated for general extended wear (see Fig. 3.1). Better safety can be assumed with the disposable system. Intolerance of solution chemicals, intolerance of hard lenses, and the need for convenience are also indications.

The lenses are contraindicated in the presence of moderate and high astigmatism.

PRESCRIBING DISPOSABLE LENSES

Fitting Acuvue lenses is done in the same manner as other soft lenses. The fitting goal is to have the lens centered so that the cornea is completely covered by the lens. Movement of approximately 0.5 mm upon blinking with the eyes in the primary position is optimal. Movement upon upgaze should be greater. The lens tends to appear slightly loose upon initial insertion, as is the case with other lenses of similar water content, but the lens will settle after being on the eye a short period of time. The lens usually reaches maximal firmness on the eye after a day; however, because disposable lenses are worn for only a week or two, the tightening that might come about with longer periods of use is not present. In addition, the increase in lens movement that sometimes results from adherence between the upper lid and the front surface of a lens with deposits is precluded because of the continuous replacement feature of disposable lenses.

Although over-refraction results with most soft lenses are variable, the excellent optical properties of the Acuvue lens require more precise spherical over-refraction. Since the lenses are not reused, it is economically beneficial to avoid the need for changes due to incorrect refraction (see Fig. 3.2). The fact that the

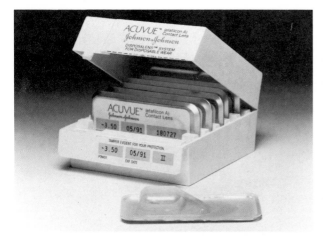

Fig. 3.1 *The disposable-lens primary and secondary package. The secondary multipack contains six lenses in individual packages. Each lens is immersed in sterile buffered saline solution. Both the primary and secondary packages are tamper-evident.*

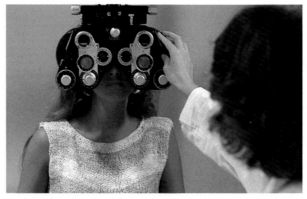

Fig. 3.2 *Refractions performed over a disposable lens must be done with care. A lens that is 0.25 diopter too strong or too weak will cause more problems for the patient than might exist with a regular hydrogel lens.*

optical properties are superior also provides the patient with better vision and, because the lens power is precise from one edge of the optic zone to the other, lenses that are slightly decentered do not affect the patient's acuity.

Lenses should be comfortable right from the time of insertion. If discomfort is present, it is usually the result of capturing a foreign body between the lens and the cornea. If discomfort is present upon lens insertion, the lens should be slid onto the sclera and then back to the cornea or removed, rinsed and reinserted (see Fig. 3.3).

INITIAL FITTING VISIT

At the initial fitting visit the proper-power lens should be chosen based on the patient's refractive error. After the lens equilibrates on the eye, a spherical over-refraction should be done; if necessary, a power change should be made based on the over-refraction.

It is extremely wise, in the event that another lens power is required, to remove and dispose of the first lens in front of the patient immediately upon removal (see Fig. 3.4). This will serve as a forceful lesson to the patient and will greatly help to ensure compliance with the wearing and disposal schedule you provide.

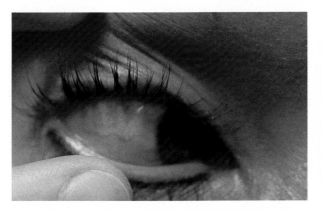

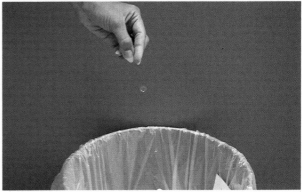

Fig. 3.3 *It is not always necessary to remove a lens from the eye if there is discomfort upon insertion. Merely sliding the lens from the cornea to the sclera and back will usually suffice. Most irritations are caused by debris or foreign bodies trapped between the lens and the cornea.*

Fig. 3.4 *When a lens is removed from the patient's eye in the examining room for any reason, it should be discarded in front of the patient. Doctors and technical staff must set proper examples.*

DISPOSABLE CONTACT LENSES

Once the proper-power lens is on, the eye movement and centration can be observed. The guiding principle regarding the physical fit of the lens should be complete corneal coverage. Lenses that are not perfectly centered but that provide complete coverage and good comfort in both the primary position and upgaze position may be prescribed confidently (see Figs. 3.5–3.7).

WEARING SCHEDULE

After 2 or 3 days of daily wear, extended wear is started. Seeing the patient on the day following the first night of extended wear

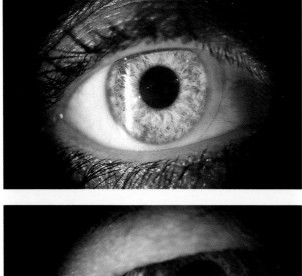

Fig. 3.5 *A perfectly centered disposable lens in place on an eye.*

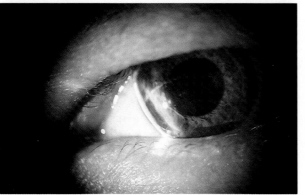

Fig. 3.6 *A more marginal fitting lens. Here the lens periphery extends beyond the limbus, but the lens is not perfectly centered. As long as the lens does not decenter enough to bare a portion of the cornea, the fit is acceptable.*

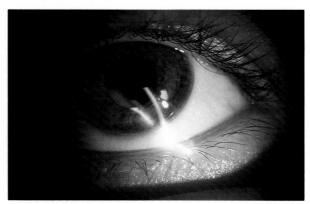

Fig. 3.7 *An unacceptable fit. In this photograph, the decentration is great enough to bare the cornea. Whenever this situation is encountered, the fitter should make certain that the lens is right side out. A lens that is inside out will frequently present this picture.*

is advisable. It is important that during the period when lenses are worn on a daily basis the patient be instructed to dispose of the lens upon removal. Again, it is necessary to set proper behavioral patterns when patients are most likely to follow instructions to the letter—that is, when they first begin wearing disposable lenses.

Most of the clinicians who worked with the lens prior to general marketing of the product prescribed 1 week extended wear, with lenses removed and thrown away before the seventh night. Patients slept without lenses on the seventh night and placed a new lens on the eye the following morning. A 1- or 2-week extended-wear schedule is used for each individual patient depending upon the judgment of the clinician.

Some clinicians believe that when a new clean lens is worn, a 2-week extended-wear schedule is warranted. These doctors, feeling that the disposable regimen provides a large increment of safety for the patient, prescribed 2-week extended wear, with lenses being removed for disposal after 14 days of wear. Patients then slept one night without lenses and put a new lens on each eye the following morning to begin another 2-week cycle.

One disadvantage to the 2-week cycle is that patients tend to remember the proper time for lens removal better when the time for removal falls on the same day each week. Obviously each clinician must choose the proper wear schedule for each patient with the above information in mind.

INSTRUCTIONS TO PATIENTS

Patients must be instructed in the proper methods for lens insertion and removal as with any other type of contact lens. In addition, some instruction about lens cleaning and disinfection is warranted. Because it is possible that a patient may have to remove a lens after an hour or two of wear in order to remove a foreign body trapped under a lens, the patient should have a small supply of cleaning, disinfecting, and saline solution. It is also extremely wise to provide written instructions for cleaning and disinfection, because patients using disposable lenses will have less practice in lens care.

Patients should also be taught to do a daily check of their own eyes using a self-monitoring triad of procedures which takes less than a minute to complete (see Fig. 3.8):

Step 1—*Feel-Good Test.* The patient should blink six to eight times; then he or she should concentrate to sense if the eyes and lenses still feel as comfortable as they usually do.

Step 2—*Look-Good-Test.* The patient should look into a mirror in a well-lighted area to check for any increase in bulbar injection and/or mucous discharge.

Step 3—*See-Well-Test.* The patient should alternately cover one eye and then the other while observing a distant picture or calendar to be sure that visual acuity is still sharp in each eye.

Patients should be instructed to take the proper action if they fail any of the tests.

In general, patients who use a continuous lens-replacement system will require fewer follow-up visits than other lens wearers. Still, a newly enrolled patient should leave the office with a thorough understanding of the recommended follow-up schedule. On return visits, it is important to check not only corneal

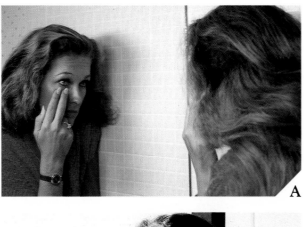

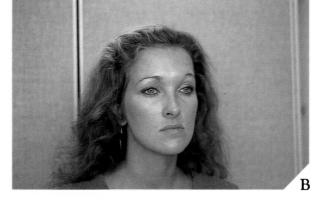

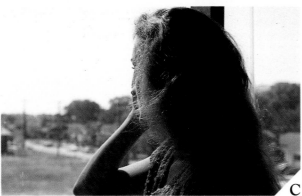

Fig. 3.8 *The self-monitoring triad. One good method to ensure that patients monitor themselves for symptoms and signs of infection is to have them determine* (A) *that the eyes are clear,* (B) *that there is no undue irritation or pain, and* (C) *that they see well each morning.*

health and visual acuity but also the patient's understanding of lens care and use. Patients who comply require fewer problem visits because they encounter fewer eye problems. A well-informed and well-managed patient will be less likely to encounter contact lens complications.

STAFF EDUCATION

Staff members should understand the key issues about disposable-lens patient care. The key points to stress to staff members are: discarding the lens after the prescribed period of use, no cleaning or reinserting, no stretching of the prescribed wear schedule, regular follow-up visits, and consultation in case of problems.

Staff members should be alert to remarks indicating that a patient is not properly following instructions. When remarks are made to a staff member indicating, for instance, that lens wear has been stretched, the staff member should be instructed to reply with the appropriate gentle criticism.

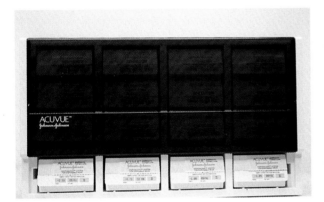

Fig. 3.9 *Office inventory modular unit for disposable lenses. Six units are shown. Each unit holds 16 multipacks (96 lenses).*

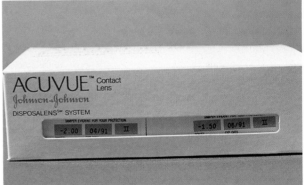

Fig. 3.10 *Disposable lenses are shipped in a box that can be used for mailing to the patient. A mailing label is included with the practitioner's return address and the patient's mailing address. Lenses can also be shipped direct to the patient from the manufacturer with the practitioner's return address.*

DISPOSABLE CONTACT LENSES

THE DISPOSALENS SYSTEM

Lenses are provided in individual plastic packages (rather than the traditional vials) encased in multipacks containing six lenses each. Each individual plastic package contains one Acuvue lens immersed in buffered saline solution. The tamper-evident individual packages are not resealable. Six individual packages are stored in each multipack, which is protected by a tamper-evident seal (see Fig. 3.9).

Clinicians are urged to enroll patients in the system for 1 year at a time. After the initial fitting, subsequent lens shipments will be sent either to the doctor's office for dispensing to the patient from the office, to the doctor's office in a box that is appropriate for reshipment to the patient, or, at the doctor's request, directly to the patient (see Fig. 3.10).

COST CONSIDERATIONS

Because of the manufacturing process, Acuvue lenses can be produced at a cost that allows disposability. Although patients still must pay a premium, the convenience, comfort, and safety advantages of continuous lens replacement are strong reasons for the additional expense. Furthermore, patients are spared the additional cost of lens care solutions and insurance policies inherent in other contact lens regimens. If one also considers that regular contact lens patients normally replace two to three lenses per year, the continuous lens-replacement system is comparably priced.

ADVANTAGES OF DISPOSABLE LENSES

Deposits, patient compliance with instructions, and patient hygiene are three of the major reasons for problems with extended-wear eye care. Although it does not solve all of the problems associated with contact lens wear, disposability does attack these major reasons for problems.

It is now well known that deposits begin to form on the front surface of lenses as soon as the lenses are applied to the eye (1–4). It is also known that even the most stringent cleaning cannot remove all deposits from the lens. The result is that as lenses are worn days, weeks, and months, they build up harmful deposits—even with the best lens cleaning available (see Fig. 3.11). This jeopardizes not only the quality of vision but also the safety of the cornea by serving as a site for the growth of bacteria and other pathogenic organisms (5,6).

Because extended-wear lenses are generally left in the eye for 2 weeks or more, they have been linked with stress to corneal phys-

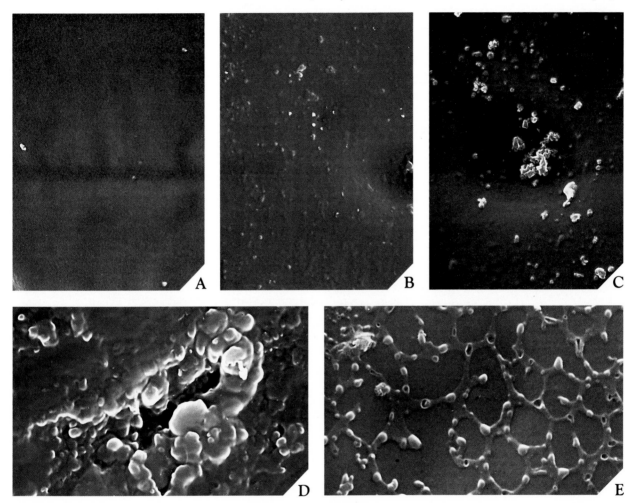

Fig. 3.11 *Photomicrographs of lens surfaces. (A) An unworn lens (×3500). The few spots of debris in the field result from making the photomicrographs. (B) A lens worn continuously for 1 week (×2500). The lens is almost clean but shows a few scattered protein deposits and debris. (C) A lens worn continuously for 2 weeks (×3400). The lens has more protein deposits and debris. (D) A lens worn continuously for 3 weeks (×3400). The lens has prominent thick and thin patches of biofilm. (E) A lens worn continuously for 3 weeks (×3600). The lens has thick and thin patches of biofilm with bacteria within the matrix. Photos courtesy of John W. Costerton, Ph.D., University of Calgary.*

DISPOSABLE CONTACT LENSES

iology and reduced resistance to eye infections (7). Various contact lens coatings actually encourage *Pseudomonas aeruginosa* to adhere to soft contact lenses (8). By failing to use a surfactant cleaner the patient increases his or her risk for this infection, which has potentially devastating consequences (9). Even with rigorous cleaning, however, it is impossible to remove all organic and inorganic materials that adhere to the lens surface (see Fig. 3.12).

Organic deposits—including protein, lipids, pigment, and fungi—can be circulated by the tears. Other deposits—including those from lotions, creams, and oil-based makeup—can be transferred from the fingers or eyelids to the lens (6). When a lens is soiled with a base of lysozyme or other protein, it will collect other types of debris more rapidly than a clean lens. With a protein base, then, lipids, hair sprays, and various types of debris will collect on that surface more quickly. Without the protein base, however, the debris has difficulty binding to the lens surface.

Protein or coating buildups, as well as clumps of deposits, on the front surface of lenses may trigger an immune response that results in giant papillary conjunctivitis (GPC) (10). Even with careful management of extended-wear patients, about half will

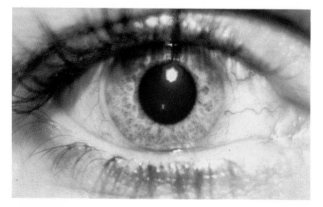

Fig. 3.12 *Adherence of organic and inorganic materials to the lens surface. Photo courtesy of Joseph F. Molinari, O.D.*

develop GPC, either from such buildups or as a result of a faulty lens edge or the poor condition of the lens (see Fig. 3.13).

Although researchers agree that an immune response exists with all contact lens wear, a greater degree is associated with extended wear because of deposits. Thorough cleaning and frequent replacement reduce the problems, but continuous replacement avoids the greatest number of infections and irritations (11,12).

Patient compliance is another major cause of problems with all contact lens patients (13–20). Noncompliant patients can fall into one of three groups: (i) those who would normally comply but are confused by the complex instructions and large number of lens care products available (see Fig. 3.14); (ii) those who are noncompliant because of laziness; and (iii) those who are noncompliant because they feel they know better than their doctor.

For confused noncompliant patients the disposable lens system is an answer to their problem. The instructions are simple. Merely remember when to remove and dispose of the lenses, and the following morning open the package and place the lenses on the eyes. There is no need to remember which solution to use for which purpose. Because the lenses are packed in buffered saline solution, it is not even necessary to decide which of a number of bottles on the dressing room shelf contains saline solution. For the patient who wants to comply but is confused by the complexity of instructions, this system is the answer.

For the lazy noncompliant patient the disposable regimen is also an answer to the problem. The system requires only (a)

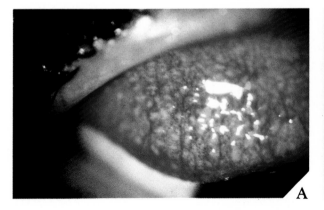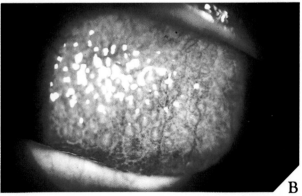

Fig. 3.13 *Giant papillary conjunctivitis resulting from a protein or coating buildup on the front* surface of a contact lens (A) or from a faulty lens edge (B).

DISPOSABLE CONTACT LENSES

removal of lenses at the appointed time and (b) replacement with a new pair of lenses the following morning. Buying solutions and washing lenses is no longer required. Disinfection, which is easily passed over, is no longer necessary. The system makes laziness a nonexistent concern.

For the patient who is noncompliant because he or she feels that the doctor is being overly careful, the disposable lens system is only a partial solution. Patients might remove and replace lenses at the prescribed time because of the convenience aspects. However, such patients might also tend to wear their lenses for longer periods because they know better than their doctor. In these cases, the patient will at least have a sterile pair of lenses to wear whenever the lenses are removed and replaced.

Although a disposable system of lens use has many advantages, it will not be a total panacea. The system does encourage compliance, and it makes complying as simple as possible. But careful personal hygiene and hygienic methods of handling lenses are required. Lenses remain sterile only as long as they remain in the original package. Once the package is opened by an un-hygienic patient the safety of the lens falls into doubt. When the lens is being placed on the eye by such a patient, it is sterile rather than merely disinfected; therefore, there will be some minimal improvement in safety.

Finally, an advantage of the disposable system is the absence of chemical disinfection solutions. Reactions to chemicals in cleaning, rinsing, and disinfecting solutions have been a problem for practitioners for several years. These problems are solved with the disposable system, because there is no need for any

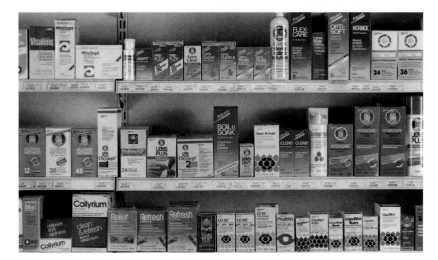

Fig. 3.14 *The large array of contact lens solutions available at any pharmacy or market may cause patients to become confused when choosing solutions.*

solution containing any of the chemicals that have been implicated in patient sensitivities. Unless something unusual happens to require rinsing or cleaning when a new lens is not available, no chemical solutions are required.

CONCLUSION

Twelve years ago, Ellis Gruber, M.D. hypothesized about a more advanced lens that could eliminate some of the problems that have plagued lens wearers all along (21):

> *If the lens could be much less costly, one could conceive of having them disposable so they could be bought in a "six-pack" and the patient could always have some on hand. The doctor could write a prescription stating "repeat as needed." The patient would then not have to worry about cleaning, or loss, or insurance premiums.*

That disposable system is now available.

REFERENCES

1. Fowler, S. A., and Allansmith, M. R. Evolution of soft contact lens coatings. *Arch. Ophthalmol.*, 98:95–99, 1980.
2. Fowler, S. A., and Allansmith, M. R. The surface of the continuously worn contact lens. *Arch. Ophthalmol.*, 98:1233–1236, 1980.
3. Sibley, M. J. Cleaning solutions for contact lenses. *Int. Contact Lens Clin.*, 9:291–294, 1982.
4. Refojo, M. F., and Holly, J. F. Tear protein absorption on hydrogels: A possible cause of contact lens allergy. *Contact Intraocul. Lens Med. J.*, 3:23–35, 1977.
5. Fowler, S. A., Greiner, J. V., and Allansmith, M. R. Attachment of bacteria to soft contact lenses. *Arch. Ophthalmol.*, 97:659–660, 1979.
6. Tripathi, R. C., Tripathi, B. J., and Ruben, M. The pathology of soft contact lens spoilage. *Am. J. Ophthalmol.*, 87:365–380, 1980.

7. Weissman, B. A. Results of the extended wear contact lens survey of the contact lens section of the american optometric association. *JAOA*, 58:159, 1987.

8. Slusher, M. M., Myrvik, Q. N., Lewis, J. C., and Gristina, A. G. Extended-wear lenses, biofilm and bacterial adhesion. *Arch. Ophthalmol.*, 105:110–115, 1987.

9. Bartlett, J. D. Are extended wear lenses safe? *JAOA*, 58:159, 1987.

10. Allansmith, M. R., Korb, D. R., Greiner, J. V., et al. Giant papillary conjunctivitis in contact lens wearers. *Am. J. Ophthalmol.*, 83:697–708, 1977.

11. Sposato, P. Excerpts from the 1987 CLAO meeting. *Contact Lens Spectrum*, 33–39, April 1987.

12. Leiblein, J. S. Benefits and risks of extended wear. *Contact Lens Forum*, 45–48, August 1986.

13. Donnenfeld, E. D., et al. Changing trends in contact lens associated corneal ulcers: An overview of 116 cases. *CLAO J.*, 12:145–149, 1986.

14. Collins, M., and Carney, L. G. Patient compliance and its influence on contact lens wearing problems. *Am. J. Optom. Physiol. Opt.*, 63:952–956, 1986.

15. Chun, M. W., and Weissman, B. A. Compliance in contact lens care. *Am. J. Optom. Physiol. Opt.*, 64:274–276, 1987.

16. Koetting, R. A., Castellano, C. F., and Wartman, R. Patient compliance with new instructions. *Contact Lens Spectrum*, 23–30, November 1986.

17. Rengstorff, R. H., Nilsson, K. T., and Sylvander, A. E. 2000 extended wear cases: A retrospective survey of contact lens complications. *J. BCLA*, 10:13–15, 1987.

18. Mondino, B. J., Weissman, B. A., Farb, M. D., and Pettit, T. H. Corneal ulcers associated with daily-wear and extended-wear contact lenses. *Am. J. Ophthalmol.*, 102:58–65, 1986.

19. Baum, J., and Boruchoff, S. A. Extended-wear contact lenses and pseudomonal corneal ulcers. *Am. J. Ophthalmol.*, 101:372–373, 1985.

20. Genvert, G. I., et al. A prospective study of emergency room visits for contact lens related problems. *CLAO J.*, 13:42–45, 1987.

21. Gruber, E. The Soflens contact lens six years later. *Contact Intraocul. Lens Med. J.*, 1:81, 1975.

4

ASTIGMATISM CORRECTION WITH RIGID CONTACT LENSES

PETER C. DONSHIK, M.D., F.A.C.S. AND
ANGELA E. LUISTRO, C.O.T., F.C.L.S.A.

The decision to use a toric lens, as well as the decision to use a specific type of toric lens, depends on the type of astigmatism that requires correction. Toric contact lenses are indicated when significant amounts of corneal toricity are present or when residual astigmatism results in poor visual acuity with a spherical contact lens. Fitting a spherical lens to a toric cornea results in a poor lens–cornea relationship and significant bearing (Fig. 4.1). Although most corneas show some toricity, a majority of patients have 2 diopters or less of corneal astigmatism. Under these circumstances, a spherical contact lens will give excellent vision and provide a satisfactory cornea–contact lens relationship. Furthermore, if smaller amounts of corneal toricity are fitted with a toric contact lens, excessive rotation will occur which will result in fluctuating vision. Therefore, one should have at least $2\frac{1}{2}$ diopters of corneal toricity to avoid this excessive rotation.

Residual astigmatism occurs when there is a significant difference between the corneal astigmatism (corneal toricity) and the refractive astigmatism (refractive cylinder). An example to illustrate the presence of a residual astigmatism would be the following case: refraction of -4.00 sphere, -2.00 cylinder, axis 180°, with keratometric readings of 43.00 at 180° by 44.00 at 90°. In this example, the refraction has a greater cylinder than is present in the keratometric readings (Fig. 4.2). There is 1 diopter of uncorrected astigmatism present, which is the residual astigmatism. A spherical lens fitted on K would manifest 1 diopter of uncorrected astigmatism. Thus, in this example, even though there is a small amount of residual astigmatism (i.e., 1 diopter), it can result in unacceptable vision when the eye is corrected with a spherical contact lens. Under these circumstances, one has to turn to a toric contact lens in order to achieve good visual acuity.

A toric lens can be defined as any lens in which one surface has two different curvatures. The surface having two different curves may be present on the anterior or front surface of the contact lens—a *front-surface toric*. If the curves are located on the posterior surface, then the design is classified as a *back-surface toric lens*. If both front and back sides of the lens have different curves, the lens is a *bitoric lens*. In addition, occasionally one can use a special aspheric design (panafocal) to correct small amounts of astigmatism that may not be corrected with a spherical lens. Although this is not truly a toric lens, it does offer an added tool to our armamentarium for fitting astigmatic individuals with gas-permeable rigid lenses.

ASTIGMATISM CORRECTION WITH RIGID CONTACT LENSES

PANAFOCAL

A *panafocal* is an aspheric front-surface contact lens. This lens is helpful in correcting residual astigmatism of less than 1 diopter. Although the amount of uncorrected residual astigmatism remains the same, the aspheric curve of the panafocal lens masks the astigmatism, thus allowing clearer visual images. This is similar to the way a thicker soft contact lens masks small amounts of residual astigmatism and achieves better visual acuity than that obtained with a thin-membrane soft contact lens. A panafocal lens is best fitted with trial lenses. Since this is not a toric contact lens, the keratometric readings should reveal less than 2 diopters of corneal toricity with a residual astigmation of 1 diopter or less. The contact lens is fitted with a trial lens on K or slightly steeper than K. As with fitting any contact lens, the lens must center and have adequate movement. An over-refraction is then performed. The lens power is calculated by adding one-half of the over-refracted cylinder to the spherical power obtained. Example: A trial lens has a base curve of 7.50 with a power of −2.00 diopters. The lens is adequately fitted so that the base curve is correct. The over-refraction is −0.50 −1.00 axis 90°, which results in 20/20 vision. Thus, the lens to order has a base curve of 7.50 with a power of −3.00 diopters (−0.50 sphere plus one-half of −1.00 equals −1.00 diopters

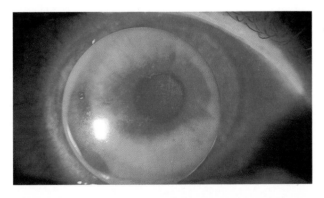

Fig. 4.1 *Spherical lens on a toric cornea showing bearing zone with corneal irritation.*

RESIDUAL ASTIGMATISM

Refraction

−4.00 −2.00 × 180° = 2 diopter cylinder

Keratometry

43.00 × 180°/44.00 × 90° = 1 diopter cylinder

Fig. 4.2 *Residual astigmatism. Comparison of refractive cylinder and corneal cylinder shows 1 diopter of difference. This difference equals the residual amount of cylinder.*

added to the -2.00 diopters of the trial lens) (Table 4.1). Because of the additional power necessary, the panafocal design may have certain disadvantages in presbyopic or pre-presbyopic individuals. However, in appropriate patients, this lens may be an alternative to the more complicated toric design lenses in treating patients with small degrees of residual astigmatism.

TABLE 4.1
PANAFOCAL FITTING SUMMARY

1. Refraction and keratometry.
2. Trial-fit with a spherical lens on *K* or slightly steeper than *K*.
3. Over-refract with sphere and cylinder for best visual acuity.
4. Calculate lens power by adding one-half of the over-refracted cylinder to the spherical power obtained.

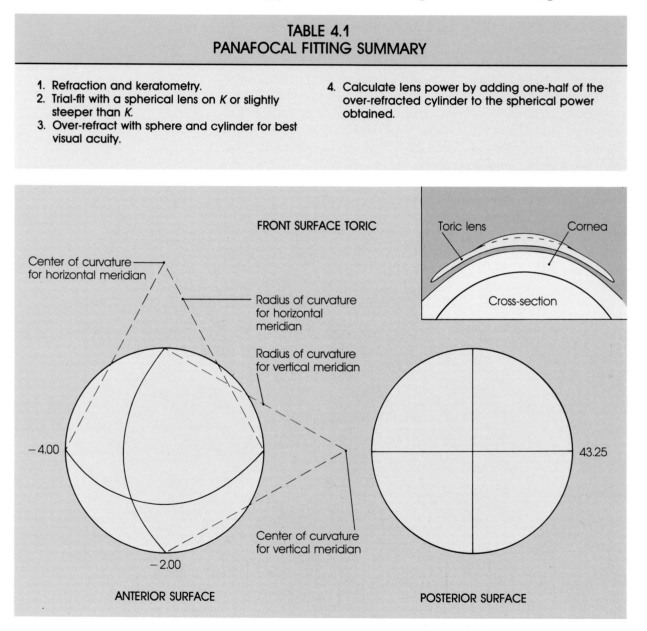

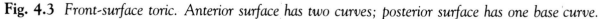

Fig. 4.3 *Front-surface toric. Anterior surface has two curves; posterior surface has one base curve.*

ASTIGMATISM CORRECTION WITH RIGID CONTACT LENSES

FRONT-SURFACE TORIC

A front-surface toric lens is a lens with a cylinder ground onto the front-surface curve. The back surface has a spherical curve (Fig. 4.3). The lens can be ordered from most laboratories and can be made from all approved gas-permeable materials. Since the cylinder correction is ground onto the front surface in one meridian, this correcting cylinder must remain at the corresponding axis to provide good visual acuity. In order to achieve this lens position, special edge designs are used to help stabilize the lens. As one blinks, lid dynamics cause the lens to rotate 10–15° nasally and to float upward before falling to the original position on the cornea. It is helpful to fit these lenses with larger diameters (9.2–9.5 mm) in order to obtain a larger optical zone. The larger optical zone will tend to decrease the noticeable fluctuation in vision that can occur with lens rotation. A prism-ballast design or a truncation design is necessary to stabilize the lens. A prism-ballast-designed lens (Figs. 4.4 and 4.5) uses a difference in thickness between the inferior aspect of the lens

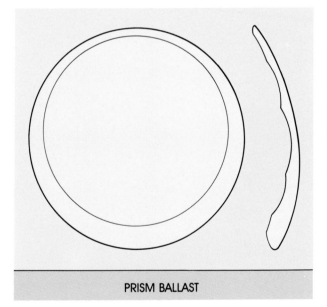

PRISM BALLAST

Fig. 4.4 *Prism ballast. Base-down prism can vary between 0.75 and 1.50 diopters.*

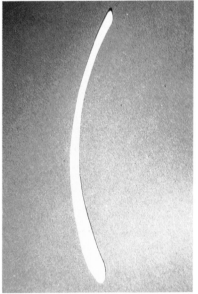

Fig. 4.5. *Photograph of a prism-ballast lens, side view (courtesy of Sola).*

(thicker) and the superior aspect of the lens (thinner) to help stabilize the lens in a given position, keeping it from rotating on the eye. The thickness of the lens base is due to the presence of prism which can vary from 0.75 diopter (minimal) to 1.5 diopters. A truncation design (Figs. 4.6 and 4.7) consists of amputating the lower part of the lens in an attempt to make the lens edge thinner without decreasing the amount of prism present. In both methods of lens stabilization, the lower edge of the lens is thicker, which can cause lens awareness and lid irritation. When fitting front-surface torics with previous rigid PMMA lenses, corneal edema is often a problem. The gas-permeable materials, because of their oxygen permeability, compensate for the increased thickness of the contact lens, thus decreasing the possibility of corneal anoxia. When these large-diameter lenses are combined with heavy prism-ballasted edges and an increase in lens thickness, tear flow can be reduced, thus creating physiological problems even though the lens material allows enough oxygen to reach the cornea. In addition, these lenses can have centration problems in that they tend to ride low with increased ocular awareness (Fig. 4.8), as compared to contact lenses with uniform thickness.

The front-surface toric lens is fitted as follows. When the corneal readings show little or no corneal toricity and the spectacle refraction contains an amount of cylinder greater than the

Fig. 4.6. *Prism truncation. Interior edge is thinned and removed to stabilize cylinder alignment.*

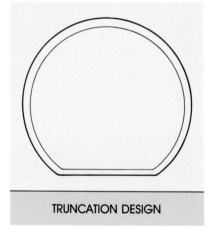

TRUNCATION DESIGN

ASTIGMATISM CORRECTION WITH RIGID CONTACT LENSES

keratometry values, a front-surface toric lens should be considered. The trial lens is a spherical lens with incorporated prism. The average amount of prism ballast is 1.25 diopters base down. The base curve of the lens should be either on K or slightly steeper than K. The starting diameter is 9.0 mm, and the spherical power of the lens should be close to the patient's spherical refraction. After the lens is inserted and settles on the patient's eye, over-refract to obtain the correct spherical power, cylinder power, and axis. Next, observe where the dot on the lens is positioned, and note the nature of the lens rotation. If the rotation is greater than 15° or 20°, the amount of prism should be increased or the truncation design may be applied to one side of the prism to counteract the rotation. If the prism amount is too small, there would be insufficient weight on the ballast to maintain proper alignment; however, too much prism may cause increased weight of the lens, resulting in patient discomfort. In ordering the final lens, the laboratory should be told of the prism alignment and amount of rotation in addition to the sphere, cylinder power, and axis. The laboratory or the fitter may determine the necessary compensation that can be expected from lid forces. Example: If the right eye is fitted with a trial lens of −3.00 diopters and over-refraction is plano −1.25 axis 90°, before ordering the final lens the amount of rotation has to be

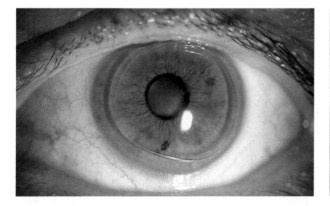

Fig. 4.7 *Photograph of a prism-truncation contact lens.*

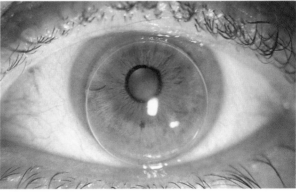

Fig. 4.8 *Front-surface toric with a prism ballast, lens riding low.*

determined. For example (Fig. 4.9), if the right lens rotates 10° nasally (to the observer's right), a lens having a 90° axis would align at an axis of 100°, thus distorting visual acuity. In order to realign the axis of the correcting cylinder, 10° has to be subtracted from the over-refracted axis. In the above example,

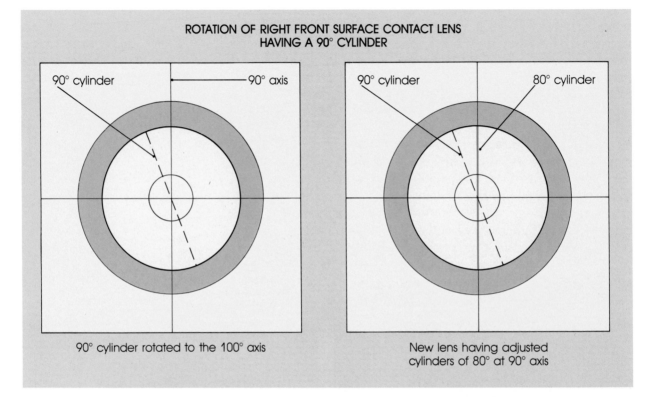

ROTATION OF RIGHT FRONT SURFACE CONTACT LENS
HAVING A 90° CYLINDER

90° cylinder — 90° axis

90° cylinder rotated to the 100° axis

90° cylinder — 80° cylinder

New lens having adjusted cylinders of 80° at 90° axis

Fig. 4.9 *Rotation of right front-surface toric contact lens. Left-hand diagram shows the dotted prism base positioned 10° to the right, which placed the effective cylinder power at 100°.*

Right-hand diagram shows the new contact lens having an 80° cylinder, which still positions 10° to the right, now placing the correcting cylinder power at 90°.

Fig. 4.10 *Front-surface toric contact lens with nasal rotation—right eye.*

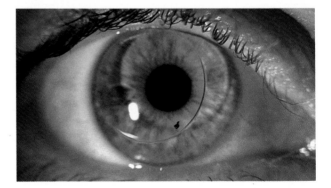

ASTIGMATISM CORRECTION WITH RIGID CONTACT LENSES

if one orders the axis at 80°, the 10° rotation will align the axis at the correct 90° meridian. It is helpful to refer to the acronym LARS, which stands for left add, right subtract. That is, if the lens rotates to the left (Fig. 4.11) the amount of rotation is added to the over-refracted axis, whereas if it rotates to the right the amount is then subtracted (Fig. 4.10) from the axis (Table 4.2). Because all prism-ballasted lenses will behave differently

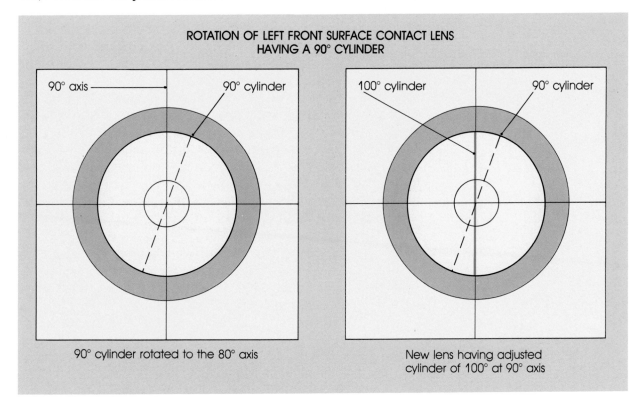

ROTATION OF LEFT FRONT SURFACE CONTACT LENS
HAVING A 90° CYLINDER

90° axis —————
90° cylinder

100° cylinder
90° cylinder

90° cylinder rotated to the 80° axis

New lens having adjusted
cylinder of 100° at 90° axis

Fig. 4.11 *Rotation of left front-surface toric contact lens.*

TABLE 4.2
FRONT-SURFACE TORIC FITTING SUMMARY

1. Refraction and keratometry.
2. Fit with a prism-ballasted trial lens having a base curve corresponding to the flattest *K*.
3. Power of trial lens should be similar to refraction.
4. Diameter of trial lens should be approximately 9.0.
5. After $\frac{1}{2}$ hr, over-refract for correct sphere, cylinder, and axis.
6. Observe lens rotation for amount and direction.
7. Compute final lens power including compensation for lens rotation.
8. Left = *add*, and Right = *subtract*, the degree of lens rotation (LARS).

on different corneas, the fitting must be done with trial lenses having the prism ballast incorporated. Depending on the volume of such fittings, one could either have a trial set of prism-ballasted lenses or obtain a diagnostic lens on a trial basis from the laboratory.

In addition to residual astigmatism (Table 4.3) described above, visual blurring with a spherical contact lens can also be due to (a) the differences in the meridians of the crystalline lens, (b) a tilt in the position of the lens, or (c) variations in the refractive index of the cornea, lens, or vitreous. An eccentric position or shape of the fovea in relationship to the visual axis can also result in residual astigmatism. Residual astigmatism may be induced by a warped contact lens or by a contact lens which, because it tilts and does not center properly, results in an induced astigmatism (1). A form of residual astigmatism called *pseudo-residual astigmatism* can occur when a thin spherical lens flexes during a blink. This diagnosis can be confirmed by taking K readings with the lens in place. The keratometric reading before the blink will be clear, but immediately after the blink the mires will be distorted. The distortion occurs because the flexure of the lens allows tears to pool centrally.

An uncorrected astigmatism will, for whatever reason, always result in blurred vision. Specifically, the patients complain of (a) vision that is usually worse at night, (b) blurred vision when reading, with doubling or ghosting of the letters, and (c) halos or distortion around lights. They often experience headaches or eyestrain.

TABLE 4.3
CAUSE OF RESIDUAL ASTIGMATISM

1. Lenticular astigmatism greater than corneal astigmatism.
2. Differences in the meridian of crystalline lens.
3. Opacities of the crystalline lens.
4. Tilt of crystalline lens or dislocation.
5. Refractive index variations of cornea, lens, or vitreous.
6. Eccentric position or shape of fovea.
7. Warped or tilted contact lens.
8. Flexure of thin spherical lens.

ASTIGMATISM CORRECTION WITH RIGID CONTACT LENSES

BACK-SURFACE TORIC

A back-surface toric contact lens is indicated in patients with large amounts of corneal toricity. In these cases, it would be very difficult to physically fit the cornea with a spherical lens. A back-surface toric lens has two curves on the posterior surface. One curve is fitted to match the flattest corneal curve, and the second curve is computed to arrive at the proper amount of back-surface toricity. The two posterior curves cannot be determined solely by the corneal keratometric values. Since the index of refraction of plastic ($n = 1.490$) and tears ($n = 1.336$) are different, the power of the cylinder will not be the same when a lens is fitted on a toric cornea. A lens made with a toric base curve will have a certain amount of induced cylinder because of the difference in the index of refraction of the two surfaces. Thus, the amount of cylinder created by the lacrimal layer depends on, and changes in relationship to, the two indexes of refraction. Therefore, the amount of cylinder cannot be determined by simply over-refracting the patient, since the induced cylinder is not taken into account. Generally, whatever the amount of difference in back-surface curvature, one-half of that amount will require additional correction (Fig. 4.12). One method of determining the cylinder is to use the back-surface conversion tables, which can be obtained from contact lens laboratories. The table allows one to determine the amount of power to apply

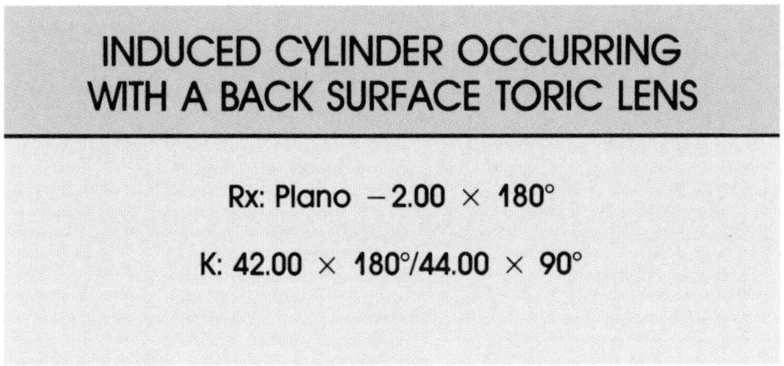

INDUCED CYLINDER OCCURRING WITH A BACK SURFACE TORIC LENS

Rx: Plano $-2.00 \times 180°$

K: $42.00 \times 180°/44.00 \times 90°$

Fig. 4.12 *Induced cylinder occurring with back-surface toric lens. If a back-surface toric is designed on K with 42.00/44.00 on the back curves, 2 diopters of toricity is generated. Approximately one-half of the back toricity is duplicated by the tear layer, giving a total astigmatism correction of 3 diopters. Since only 2 diopters of astigmatism is needed, the back-surface design has created an extra diopter of cylinder.*

to the second curvature of the toric lens (Table 4.4). An illustration of this concept follows:

K-READING	REFRACTION	FIRST CURVE FITTED ON FLAT K
42.00 × 180/45.00 × 90	− 3.50 − 2.50 × 180	= 42.00

In the above example, − 2.50 diopters of cylinder needs to be corrected. One consults the table and finds that for a − 2.50-diopter correction "in air cylinder," one needs − 1.75 diopters on the back surface of the lens for the second curvature. Therefore, one adds 1.75 to the flattest curvature (42.00) to arrive at the second curve of 43.75. The power remains unchanged, since the lens was fitted on flat K-readings (in this example, one does not have to consider vertex distance). The lens in this example that is to be ordered would be 42.00/43.75 with a power of − 3.50 diopters. The diameter should be at least 9.0 mm to help lens centration. This example fully corrects the refractive error without inducing an astigmatic effect (Table 4.5). If, however, the lens fit is inadequate or more cylinder correction is found necessary with an over-refraction, then consider a bitoric lens. Because the back-surface toric lens is difficult to fit and is not well standardized, it has fallen into some disfavor among the majority of contact lens fitters.

TABLE 4.4
BACK-SURFACE CONVERSION TABLE

In Air Cylinder (diopters)	Cylinder Back Surface (diopters)	In Air Cylinder (diopters)	Cylinder Back Surface (diopters)	In Air Cylinder (diopters)	Cylinder Back Surface (diopters)
0.50	0.25	3.25	2.25	6.25	4.25
0.75	0.50	3.75	2.50	6.50	4.50
1.00	0.75	4.00	2.75	7.00	4.75
1.50	1.00	4.25	3.00	7.25	5.00
2.00	1.25	4.75	3.25	7.50	5.25
2.25	1.50	5.00	3.50	8.00	5.50
2.50	1.75	5.50	3.75	8.25	5.75
3.00	2.00	5.75	4.00	8.75	6.00

ASTIGMATISM CORRECTION WITH RIGID CONTACT LENSES

BITORIC CONTACT LENSES

The bitoric contact lens has compound curves on both its anterior and posterior surfaces. The rules of fitting are that the flattest meridian always gets the most plus power or least minus power. The steepest meridian always gets the most minus power or the least plus power. The diameter should be in the range of 9.0–9.5 mm, which will provide good centration and positioning of the lenses. Bitoric lenses are indicated when there is at least 2.5 diopters of corneal astigmatism combined with a similar amount of refractive astigmatism. It is important to compute the refractive error in minus cylinder and make the necessary corrections for vertex distance when indicated (Table 4.6). To illustrate the fitting of bitoric lenses, the optical cross method is helpful (Vision Ease Educational Bulletin). By this method, one can analyze the refraction and corneal curvature as if they

---

TABLE 4.5
BACK-SURFACE TORIC FITTING SUMMARY

1. Refraction and keratometry.
2. Determine lens curvature by using flattest *K* for first posterior curve.
3. Use conversion table to determine second posterior curve by adding value from table to flattest *K*.
4. Power of lens in equal to refractive sphere power considering vertex distance when necessary.
5. Diameter should be at least 9.0 for good centration.

TABLE 4.6
BITORIC FITTING SUMMARY

1. Refraction and keratometry.
2. Draw two optical crosses side by side.
3. Put refraction and *K* on first optical cross, giving the flattest meridian the most plus power and the steepest meridian the most minus power.
4. Use the second optical cross to design base curve and power.
5. Fit the flattest corneal curve on *K*.
6. Fit the steepest corneal curve approximately 0.50 diopter flatter than *K*.
7. Make any necessary vertex changes.
8. Take the base curve and power from the second optical cross, convert back to Rx for power.
9. Diameter should be 9.0–9.5

---

were two spherical entities. An example to illustrate this is the following:

REFRACTION   K-READING

+2.00 −3.00 × 180   42.00 × 180/45.00 × 90

The above example can be considered to consist of one sphere with a +2.00 diopter power at 180° and a second sphere with a −1.00 diopter power at 90°, as seen in Fig. 4.13. The rule is that the steepest meridian always gets the most minus or the least plus. Here the steepest meridian is at 90° and should get the most minus power. However, in designing the lens curvature, the vertical meridian should be fitted slightly flatter (approximately 0.50 diopters) than the vertical keratometry readings in order to enhance tear circulation and to get a better fit. Therefore, adjustments are made on a second optical cross in the vertical meridian, as shown in Fig. 4.14. The 180° meridian has a +2.00-diopter power with a curvature of 42.00, and the ver-

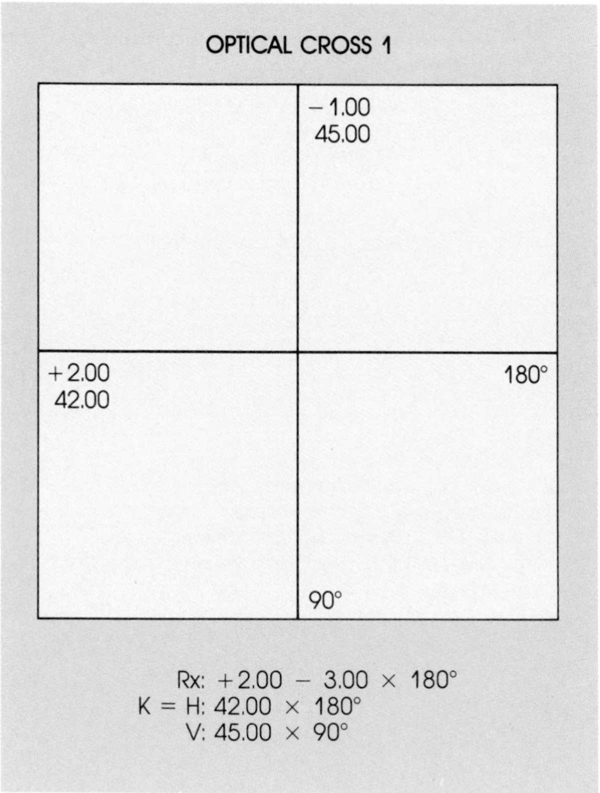

Fig. 4.13 *Optical cross 1 (+2.00 −3.00 × 180°). Add the sphere and cylinder, and give the total power to the vertical meridian. The horizontal meridian is given the power of the spherical portion of the refraction.*

OPTICAL CROSS 1

−1.00
45.00

+2.00
42.00

180°

90°

Rx: +2.00 − 3.00 × 180°
K = H: 42.00 × 180°
V: 45.00 × 90°

ASTIGMATISM CORRECTION WITH RIGID CONTACT LENSES

tical meridian now has a power of -0.50 at 44.50 (0.5 diopter of plus had to be added to the power to compensate for the 0.5-diopter flatter curvature). The base curve of the lens to be ordered is depicted in Fig. 4.14 using the second optical cross (42.00/44.50). Next convert the power to a spectacle Rx (subtract sphere and cylinder algebraically), which in this example gives a value of $+2.00 - 2.50$. It is not necessary to specify the axis because the lens will seek its own alignment on the eye. The final lens that will be ordered (for this example) has base

Fig. 4.14 *Optical cross 2 ($+2.00 - 3.00 \times 180°$).*

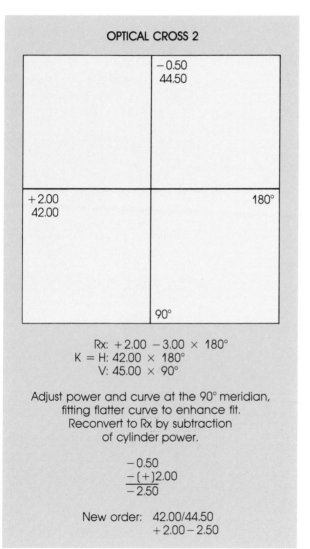

OPTICAL CROSS 2

-0.50
44.50

$+2.00$
42.00

180°

90°

Rx: $+2.00 - 3.00 \times 180°$
K = H: $42.00 \times 180°$
V: $45.00 \times 90°$

Adjust power and curve at the 90° meridian,
fitting flatter curve to enhance fit.
Reconvert to Rx by subtraction
of cylinder power.

-0.50
$-(+)2.00$
$\overline{-2.50}$

New order: 42.00/44.50
$+2.00 - 2.50$

curves of 42.00/44.50, a power of $+2.00 -2.50$ diopters. You must make sure that the labs know that you have reconverted the power to the actual spectacle refraction and are not taking the power directly off the optical cross, which would be $+2.00$ -0.50. An illustration of this follows:

REFRACTION	K-READING
$+4.50 -2.75 \times 010$	$41.50 \times 10/44.50 \times 100$ [Fig. 4.15 (optical cross 3) and Fig. 4.16 (optical cross 4)]

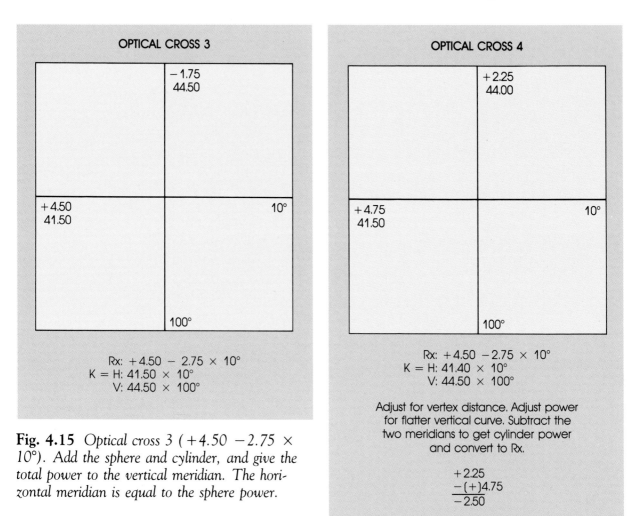

OPTICAL CROSS 3

-1.75
44.50

$+4.50$
41.50

$10°$

$100°$

Rx: $+4.50 - 2.75 \times 10°$
K = H: $41.50 \times 10°$
V: $44.50 \times 100°$

Fig. 4.15 *Optical cross 3 ($+4.50 -2.75 \times 10°$). Add the sphere and cylinder, and give the total power to the vertical meridian. The horizontal meridian is equal to the sphere power.*

OPTICAL CROSS 4

$+2.25$
44.00

$+4.75$
41.50

$10°$

$100°$

Rx: $+4.50 -2.75 \times 10°$
K = H: $41.40 \times 10°$
V: $44.50 \times 100°$

Adjust for vertex distance. Adjust power for flatter vertical curve. Subtract the two meridians to get cylinder power and convert to Rx.

$$+2.25$$
$$\underline{-(+)4.75}$$
$$-2.50$$

New order: $41.50/44.00$
$+4.75-2.50$

Fig. 4.16 *Optical cross 4 ($+4.50 - 2.75 \times 10°$).*

Bitoric lenses usually center and move well because of the close lens–cornea relationship. If a lens does not center properly, consider increasing the lens diameter. If it still rides high or decenters, it may be too flat. A low-positioned lens may be a result of incomplete blinking or a steep fit. The lens diameter may be decreased in order to flatten the lens–cornea relationship. If the lens is still too flat or too steep, readjust the curves and obtain the correct power by recalculating them via the optical cross method previously discussed.

LENS FLEXURE

In some situations, lens flexure (Fig. 4.17) can cause problems in the contact lens correction of visual acuity. As a general rule, lens flexure can induce astigmatism in the absence of corneal toricity and can mask astigmatism in the presence of corneal toricity. To determine when flexure will either be a problem or an advantage, compare the refractive cylinder and the keratometry cylinder. If the refraction is $-1.50 -1.50 \times 180$ and the keratometric value is $44.00 \times 5/45.25 \times 90$, then the refractive cylinder is within 0.5 diopter of the corneal cylinder, and the refractive axis is aligned with the flattest K. In this

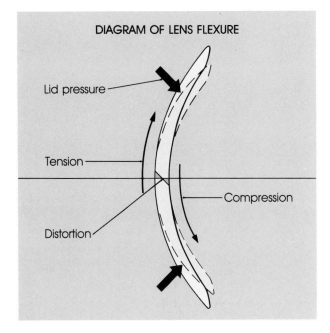

Fig. 4.17 *Diagram of lens flexure.*

ASTIGMATISM CORRECTION WITH RIGID CONTACT LENSES

example, with-the-rule astigmatism is also present. If such an eye were fitted with a thin contact lens, flexure would occur and fluctuating vision would result. Therefore, to avoid flexure, a lens with a standard center thickness (0.16 mm) rather than a thinner lens would be desirable. On the other hand, if the patient had, instead, a refraction of $-1.50 \, -0.75 \times 10$ and keratometric reading of $44.00 \times 5/45.50 \times 95$, there would be a greater amount of cylinder on the cornea than in the refraction. In this example, the refractive cylinder axis is also in the same meridian as the flatter K-readings. In this example, the potential for residual astigmatism exists and flexure would be desired. If the lens is thin enough to bend slightly during the blink cycle, most or all of the potential residual astigmatism will be corrected. A thin gas-permeable lens with an average center thickness of 0.12 mm would be indicated.

In summary, it is easiest to remember that when the refraction and K-readings are similar, use a standard thickness to prevent flexure; however, when the corneal toricity is greater, use thinner lenses to allow flexure to occur, and this may help improve the vision. An exception to this rule would be a distorted corneal reading. Some practitioners attempt to compensate for lens flexure on a toric cornea by fitting slightly flatter than K when with-the-rule astigmatism is present and by fitting slightly steeper when against-the-rule astigmatism is present, instead of changing the center thickness of the lens.

SUMMARY

Toric designs are useful in our armamentarium for correction of the astigmatic refractive error. They have been available since the early days of rigid contact lens fittings. However, they are more attractive today because of the ability to manufacture toric lenses in gas-permeable materials. Although fitting these lenses in the past has caused certain compromises with regard to corneal physiology, the gas-permeable polymers have enabled many of these physiologic problems to be resolved. We have a variety of toric designs to fit the different types of astigmatic refractive errors that are present in our contact lens patients. The ability to utilize toric design lenses will increase our ability to fit a large number of patients who desire contact lenses.

REFERENCES

1. Polseka, Kenyon E. Special refractive problems. In: Aquavella, J. V., and Rao, G. N. (Eds.), *Contact Lenses*, p. 164, J. B. Lippincott, Philadelphia, 1987.

2. Maltzman, B. A., Koeniger, E., and Dabezies, O. H. Correction of astigmatism: Hard lenses. In: Dabezies, O. H. (Ed.), *Contact Lenses: The CLAO Guide to Basic Science Clinical Practice*, Chapter 50, p. 50.8, Grune & Stratton, New York, 1984.

5
ASTIGMATISM CORRECTION WITH SOFT CONTACT LENSES

MICHAEL HARRIS, M.D.

Any practitioner who wants to offer full contact lens services must be able to fit soft toric lenses. Approximately 25% of patients will have significant astigmatism (over 1.00 diopters). Many of these patients will not tolerate the optics of spherical soft lenses or the discomfort of a rigid contact lens. These patients desire the comfort of soft lenses and the vision of spectacles.

MATERIALS AND THEORY

Soft toric lenses are manufactured by a number of major companies. They offer inventory lenses of common power and axis. Custom lenses of unusual parameters are available from these same companies. In addition, there are several smaller manufacturers who specialize in these custom lenses.

All soft torics have one thing in common: They are designed to orient in a particular position that should be stable from blink to blink and upon changes in gaze.

The various designs will be briefly described, and their advantages and disadvantages will be mentioned.

PRISM BALLAST

A contact lens with prism ballast (Fig. 5.1) is basically a lens that has been made thicker and heavier in 30–45% of its circumference. Gravity, no doubt, has some effect on the

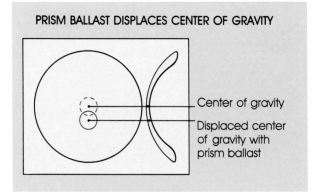

Fig. 5.1 *Prism-ballast concept.*

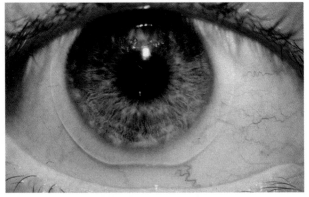

Fig. 5.2 *Truncated lens.*

orientation of the lens; but it is, to a greater degree, the uneven distribution of lens mass that accounts for the positioning. The dynamics of lid closure (which will be mentioned in greater detail in the section on rotational problems) force the heavier, thicker portion of lens along the inferior lid margin.

TRUNCATION

To truncate a lens is to shorten one side. More simply, a portion of the lens is amputated as seen in Fig. 5.2. The theory behind truncation is that the flat side of the lens will be tapped into proper place as the lens rests against the lower lid (Fig. 5.3). Truncation is usually used in conjunction with prism ballast. Investigation by Wesley Jessen, during the FDA investigational period for their lenses, showed that truncation increased lens stability over prism ballast alone.

CHAMFERING

This is a modification of the prism ballast and truncation combination. If one takes a prism-ballasted lens and then decides to truncate it, one would cut a section of lens off at *right* angles to the lens. Now if one decided to truncate a prism-ballasted lens at an oblique angle, so as to remove material and thus create a tapered lens that doesn't lose diameter, as pictured in Fig. 5.4, we would have a chamfered lens.

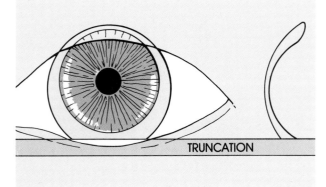

Fig. 5.3 *Truncated lens principle.*

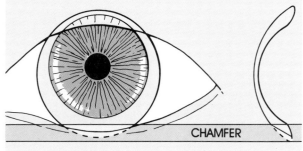

Fig. 5.4 *Chamfering principle.*

DOUBLE CHAMFERING

If truncation increases stability and if chamfering is a form of truncation, a lens could also be designed with chamfering above for the upper lid and below for the lower lid (Fig. 5.5). This lens could also be designed without prism ballast, thereby reducing lens mass without sacrificing lens diameter. This is the design of Ciba's Torisoft.

LENS DIAMETERS

All of the previously mentioned designs could be produced in any size. Experience has shown that the larger the contact, the more stable it is. The smallest effective diameter, in my opinion, is 14.0 mm. Custom toric lenses with large refractive cylindrical corrections should be 15.0 mm or greater. Presently, most lenses are 14.0–15.0 mm in diameter.

WATER CONTENT

Lenses are available in daily-wear (38–43%) and extended-wear (55% +) water contents. Results are more predictable with daily wear. The lower the water content, the more predictably the lens will behave under a variety of environmental conditions (humidity, tear supply, etc.). Also, as extended-wear lenses age, they tighten to a greater degree than daily wear, and this change in the fitting characteristics of the lens may affect the orientation of the astigmatic portion.

Economics is also a disadvantage with regard to extended-wear lenses. These lenses will need replacement sooner and will cost more both initially and for replacement.

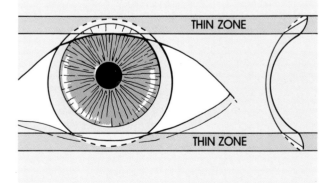

Fig. 5.5 *Double-chamfering principle.*

ASTIGMATISM CORRECTION WITH SOFT CONTACT LENSES

FRONT TORICS VERSUS BACK TORICS

Some manufacturers have chosen to place the toric surface on the posterior (inside) surface of the lens, the theory being to effect a "hand and glove" fit. The toric contact lens surface "locks" into the toric surface of the cornea. This design will work on pure corneal astigmatism but will fail to offer any greater stability and may even destabilize a lens on a toric cornea with residual astigmatism (see section on mixed residual astigmatism). However, this design is very useful with large corneal astigmatism (4–6 diopters).

A front toric lens can be used in any astigmatic situation. Because the cylinder is placed on the front surface, it can be likened to a spectacle correction, which disregards the origin of astigmatism and only regards the net refraction.

DESIGN ADVANTAGES AND DISADVANTAGES

There is *no* ideal design. Prism ballast is the mainstay of lens stability. However, a thicker edge may be a source of discomfort to many patients. (The Bausch & Lomb Optima toric minimizes this problem by dynamic distribution of lens mass, gradually increasing thickness from top to bottom of the lens. This yields an edge thickness less than normal in the upper lid area and only slightly greater than normal thickness on the lower lid surface, whereas a traditional prism-ballast lens has normal thickness above and "super-thickness" below.)

Truncation has an advantage with stability but also raises the center of gravity of the lens. This can cause some difficulty in downgaze (reading). For this reason, truncated lenses are best avoided in hyperopic prescriptions.

Chamfering is, to my mind, a better way to truncate. Double chamfering makes for an extremely comfortable lens but is less stable than prism-ballast/truncated or prism-ballast/chamfered lenses.

So, is there one lens that has superior design? The answer is no! Lens stability, patient comfort, and the *origin of the astigmatism* are going to dictate the best lens design for each individual patient.

The office fitting set should have at least four designs: a prism-ballast lens; a combo lens; a prism-ballast/truncated lens, or a prism-ballast/chamfer lens; a double-chamfered lens; and a back toric lens for large corneal astigmatism.

SOLUTIONS

Daily-wear soft toric lenses can be handled by traditional heat or cold systems. Extended-wear lenses usually require a non-thermal system.

Cleaning, with either type, must be meticulous. The collection of debris or oil on the lenses may cause them to rotate, and the prescription will be imprecise after rotation. Enzyme cleaner is encouraged.

Baking soda has been used as an adjunct to surface cleaner at my office for many years. A paste consisting of approximately four drops of daily cleaner and a "pinch" of baking soda is employed. (The easiest way to obtain the right consistency is to wet the tip of one's index finger and stick one's finger into the box of baking soda.) The baking soda that sticks to the finger is then rubbed into the lens, which is held in the palm with four drops of daily cleaner already added. This yields a mildly gritty suspension. The lens is rubbed vigorously on both sides and is then rinsed with saline. Baking soda alkalinizes the material, making it more hydrophilic. It is bacteriostatic and mechanically removes oils and makeup.

ASSESSMENT OF ASTIGMATISM

CONVENTIONS AND NOTATION

1. *K*-READINGS. All *K*-readings will be expressed using the following convention:

K = Flattest *K*/steepest *K* × Axis of steeper *K*

EXAMPLE: *K* = 42/44 × 180

This convention removes any confusion when dealing with oblique astigmatism. It is also easier to correlate to refractions when *plus cylinder* is used.

EXAMPLE: *K* = 42/44 × 180 and patient's Rx = +2.00 + 2.00 × 180

2. REFRACTION. In assessing astigmatism, we use the following notation:

F = refraction

F_a = automated refraction

F_c = cycloplegic refraction

F_m = manifest refraction

TYPES OF ASTIGMATISM

The types of astigmatism are as follows: pure corneal astigmatism; pure lenticular astigmatism; mixed favorable astigmatism; mixed residual astigmatism; and irregular astigmatism. These will be discussed in the following subsections.

PURE CORNEAL ASTIGMATISM

This situation exists when all the astigmatism, determined by cycloplegic or automated refraction, equals the toricity of the cornea.

EXAMPLE: $K = 41/45 \times 90$

$F_a = -2.00 + 4.00 \times 90$

PURE LENTICULAR ASTIGMATISM

This situation exists when all the astigmatism, determined by cycloplegic or automated refraction, arises from the lens of the eye.

EXAMPLE: $K = 42$ sphere

$F_a = -2.00 + 4.00 \times 90$

MIXED FAVORABLE ASTIGMATISM

This situation arises when the corneal astigmatism and the lenticular astigmatism balance to net no astigmatism, as determined by refraction.

EXAMPLE: $K = 42/43.50 \times 90$

$F_c = -2.00$ sphere

MIXED RESIDUAL ASTIGMATISM

This situation arises when there is both corneal and lenticular astigmatism and the axes of the meridians are located differently, resulting in a vector resultant astigmatism.

In the following example, the amount of corneal and lenticular astigmatism is equal but at a different axis. The resulting astigmatism, found during refraction, is different than the meridian measured separately on the cornea.

EXAMPLE: $K = 41/45 \times 90$

$\qquad F_c = -2.00 + 4.00 \times 30$

A variant of mixed residual astigmatism would be that the cylinder axis of the refraction and the cornea are the same, but the amount of astigmatism is different. A lenticular astigmatism exists that only partially negates the corneal astigmatism.

EXAMPLE: $K = 41/45 \times 90$

$\qquad F_c = -2.00 + 1.50 \times 90$

Other variants would combine the two previous examples.

IRREGULAR ASTIGMATISM
This type of astigmatism is the result of pathology in the cornea: keratoconus, corneal scarring, pterygium, corneal warpage syndrome, status post-refractive surgery. *Toric soft* lenses *are not recommended for these conditions.*

LENS SELECTION WITH REGARD TO ASTIGMATISM

If one now reviews the section on materials and theory as well as the section on solutions, some correlations between lens design and types of astigmatism can be made.

Back toric lenses are most useful with pure corneal astigmatism. People with very high astigmatism usually have pure corneal astigmatism. It is for this reason that custom-made lenses for astigmatism greater than 2 diopters are usually back toric. The resultant "hand and glove" fit is very stable. These lenses are usually 15.0 mm in diameter to enhance stability.

Front toric lenses correct any astigmatic refractive problems, but don't address the source of the astigmatism, and stability is based on the other elements of lens design, prism ballast, etc.

My recommendation is to use front-toric-designed lenses for astigmatism of 1–2 diopters and to use back-toric-designed lenses for high astigmatic patients.

ROTATIONS

In performing a fitting, the K-readings are taken, the astigmatism is analyzed, and a lens is selected. All toric lenses have markings on them. Some have a dot or hash markings at the 6 o'clock position; others have horizontal hash markings. If the lens has been ordered with the axis of the cylinder at the same axis as the refraction, the lens will work *if and only if* the dot is at 6 o'clock (give or take 5–10°). If there is more rotation than this, the vision will be blurred. The smaller the cylinder ordered, the less significant a rotation will be. The larger the cylinder, the more disastrous a distortion the rotation will cause (Fig. 5.6).

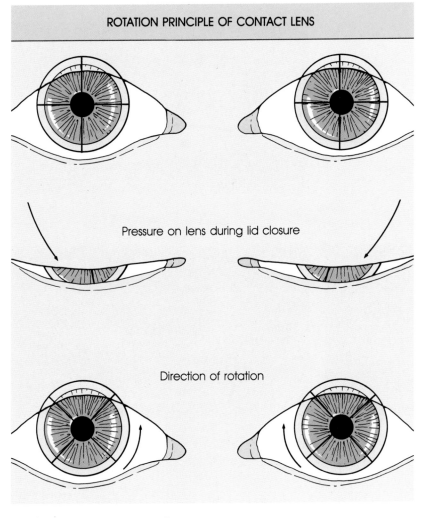

ROTATION PRINCIPLE OF CONTACT LENS

Pressure on lens during lid closure

Direction of rotation

Fig. 5.6 *Rotation principle.*

WHY DO ROTATIONS OCCUR?

There are several forces at work to disrupt good lens alignment.

LID CONTOUR (FIG. 5.7)

Rarely will one find a perfectly horizontal lower lid as shown in Fig. 5.8. Some lids slant mongoloid or antimongoloid. Lids have differing amounts of scleral coverage based on lid size and orbit depth.

LID CLOSURE

As shown in Fig. 5.9, the lid closes lateral to medial as well as up and down (Figs. 5.10 and 5.11). This action, which has been called the "zipper effect" of lid closure, facilitates moving the

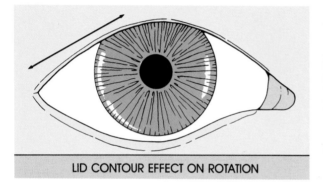

Fig. 5.7 *Lid contour effect on rotation.*

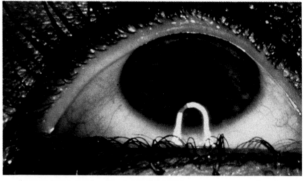

Fig. 5.8 *Lid contour—horizontal lid.*

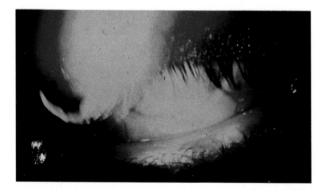

Fig. 5.9 *Normal lid closure (from temporal to nasal).*

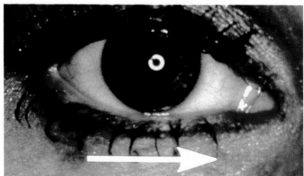

Fig. 5.10 *Normal lid closure (from temporal to nasal).*

ASTIGMATISM CORRECTION WITH SOFT CONTACT LENSES

tear film to the medial canthus. However, these forces cause a counterclockwise rotation of a contact lens.

ROTATIONS RELATED TO IMPROPER FIT

If a lens is fitted properly, the base curve selected gives a well-centered lens (Fig. 5.12), with 1–2 mm of movement on a blink, and a slight downward lag movement on upgaze (Fig. 5.13). As stated in the previous section, the position of the lens may be slightly rotated off-axis, but it must be stable (Fig. 5.14).

Two types of rotations will be seen with lenses that are fit too loosely or too tightly. Lenses that are grossly too tight or loose are easily diagnosed.

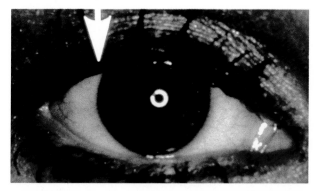

Fig. 5.11 *Normal lid closure (from up to down).*

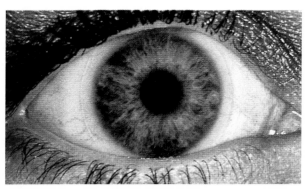

Fig. 5.12 *Well centering of lens.*

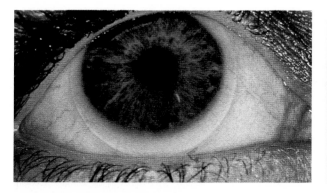

Fig. 5.13 *Well centering of lens—normal 1–2-mm vertical lag movement with blink.*

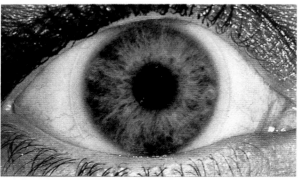

Fig. 5.14 *Well centering of lens—normal return to centered position.*

GROSSLY TIGHT LENS (Fig. 5.15)

Poor vision

Good initial comfort that degrades in hours

Red eye

Limbal impression of lens edge

Difficult to dislodge from cornea

Trapped air bubbles

GROSSLY LOOSE LENS

Decentered in position, usually upward (Fig. 5.16)

Excessive movement after a blink (Fig. 5.17)

Initial comfort poor and gets worse

Easily dislodged from cornea

Edge standoff (Fig. 5.18)

Occasionally, a lens will look like a good fit but will demonstrate an unstable rotation.

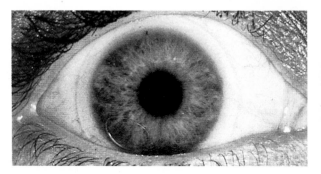

Fig. 5.15 *Tight lens with bubble, scleral indentation, conjunctival drag, and capillary blanching.*

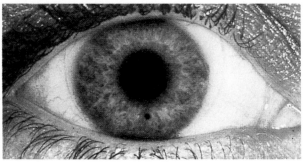

Fig. 5.16 *Loose lens with upward decentration.*

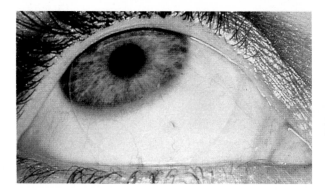

Fig. 5.17 *Loose lens with excessive movement after blink.*

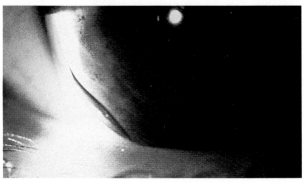

Fig. 5.18 *Loose lens with edge flexing (stand off) at lower lid margin.*

CREEPING ROTATION (TIGHT LENS)

On each successive blink the lens will move counterclockwise incrementally (Fig. 5.19). These lenses will usually rotate 50–60° before they come to rest, and then they will become more and more uncomfortable. This is the result of a minimally tight lens which moves in response to lid forces but which is too tight to recorrect itself by its design (prism ballast, truncation, etc.) and come back to its original position. See Figs. 5.20–5.22, where the normal dot has been accentuated with india ink, for purposes of demonstration.

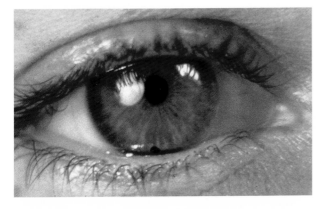

Fig. 5.19 *Normal counterclockwise movement (creeping lens rotation) with blink.*

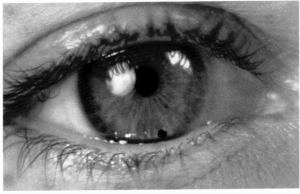

Fig. 5.20 *Normal counterclockwise movement (creeping lens rotation) with blink.*

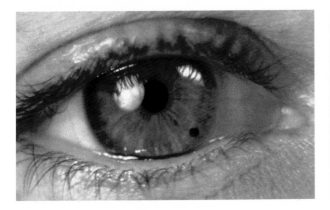

Fig. 5.21 *Normal counterclockwise movement (creeping lens rotation) with blink.*

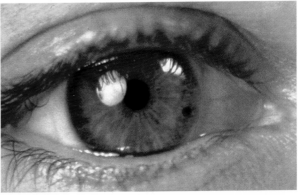

Fig. 5.22 *Normal counterclockwise movement (creeping lens rotation) with blink.*

ERRATIC ROTATIONS (LOOSE LENS)

In this unstable rotation (as shown in Figs. 5.23–5.26), upon successive blinking, the lens will move left or right of its intended position, and vision will fluctuate accordingly. In this situation, the eye-care specialist should reorder the lens with a steeper base curve.

CORRECTING THE RX FOR A STABLE ROTATION

Unstable (creeping or erratic) rotations should be corrected by refitting (Figs. 5.27 and 5.28). Stable rotations can be compensated for by adjusting the cylinder axis of the contact lens. Do this if the adjustment will be up to 20° of change. Adjustments larger than this will cause such a change in the lens' characteristics that it will not predictably rotate as it did before the adjustment was made. A better solution would be to choose a different manufacturer's lens which one knows to be more stable in design.

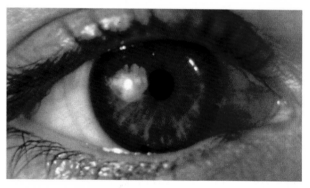

Fig. 5.23 *Erratic lens rotation.*

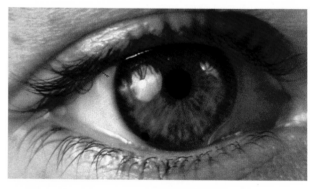

Fig. 5.24 *Erratic lens rotation.*

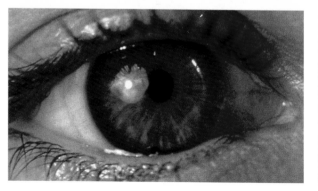

Fig. 5.25 *Erratic lens rotation.*

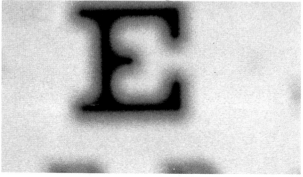

Fig. 5.26 *Erratic lens rotation.*

ASTIGMATISM CORRECTION WITH SOFT CONTACT LENSES

MNEMONIC FOR CORRECTING SMALL STABLE ROTATIONS—LARS (LEFT ADD, RIGHT SUBTRACT)

The mnemonic states the following: If the axis rotates to the examiner's left, and the lens Rx is written in *minus cylinder*, the adjustment is made by subtracting the amount of estimated rotation from the Rx (Figs. 5.29–5.31).

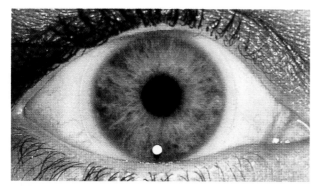

Fig. 5.27 *Axis moves away from stable position after blink.*

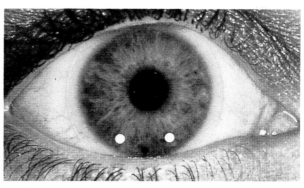

Fig. 5.28 *Dot stabilizes in the 90° base-down position.*

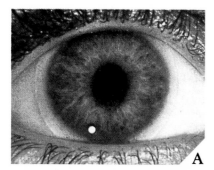

A

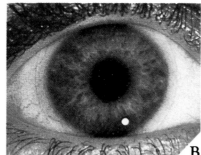

B

Fig. 5.29 (A) *Left add,* (B) *right subtract (LARS).*

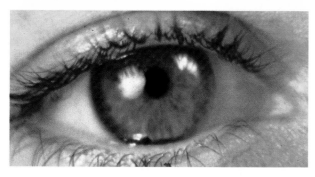

Fig. 5.30 *Estimating drift angle.*

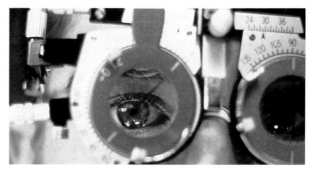

Fig. 5.31 *Drift-angle measurement technique.*

EXAMPLE: Rx: $-2.00 - 1.50 \times 90$

            LARS: Dot 15° to the left (left add)

           Order: $-2.00 - 1.50 \times 105$

And, similarly, if the lens rotates to the examiner's right, the amount of estimated rotation, in degrees, is subtracted from the original Rx to yield the final Rx.

EXAMPLE: Rx: $-2.00 - 1.50 \times 90$

            LARS: Dot 15° to the right (right subtract)

           ORDER: $-2.00 - 1.50 \times 75$

STEPWISE FITTING

Now that one has read the sections on lens design and understands the various astigmatic types and the dynamics of stable and unstable rotations, one is ready for an organized approach to fitting. In this section, some "pearls of wisdom" will be offered to increase success.

PATIENT ASSESSMENT

1. Avoid extremely fussy patients. These are patients who can discriminate the slightest errors in their spectacles. The dynamic nature of even a good fit will stimulate more dissatisfaction in these patients than either *you* or *they* can tolerate.

2. Follow the 25 rule (Fig. 5.32), which states the following: *Select soft toric lenses for patients over 25 years of age with astigmatism who have never worn lenses.* Rarely will you find a patient over 25 years old who will adapt satisfactorily to a rigid lens, even if it is very oxygen-permeable. You can use soft toric lenses for patients under 25 years old (especially if only one eye requires astigmatic correction), but you can also consider rigid lenses or Saturn II. Do not select this lens for someone over 25 years old who has grown intolerant of hard lenses but is still adapted to

Fig. 5.32
Physiologic changes in the corneal tolerance for hypoxia rule out rigid lenses as the lens of choice, unless the patient has been wearing rigid lenses and has developed corneal adaptation.

ASTIGMATISM CORRECTION WITH SOFT CONTACT LENSES

hard lenses. Refit these patients with rigid O_2 permeable lenses. These patients are usually uncomfortable because of corneal hypoxia. The oxygen-permeable lens will correct this. Such patients will be much happier with handling and caring for a lens that is similar to what they have worn for years.

3. Avoid patients with blepharitis and dry eyes. Although these patients may be successful initially, the deposits and dehydration of their lenses will cause fitting problems weeks to months after dispensing. The lens will rotate off-axis easily if the surface friction between the lens surface and the upper tarsus is increased by dryness or deposits.

4. Avoid patients who are not willing to replace their lenses at least once a year. (For reason, see paragraph 3.)

5. Avoid patients who are wearing spherical lenses or spherical spectacles and do not improve at least two lines of Snellen acuity with the addition of cylinder. If a patient like this does want the improvement, give no more than 1.00 diopter of cylinder in the contact lens Rx.

If the patient passes the above criteria, go to the next step, namely, keratometry and refraction.

KERATOMETRY AND REFRACTION

Keratometry can be manual or automated. The refraction should be done in the same fashion as for spectacles. The automated refraction is very useful in contact lens fitting. It can be done early in the exam to analyze the astigmatism. The autorefractor simulates a cycloplegic refraction without using drops. However, for ordering a contact lens Rx, I prefer not to "cyclopleg" the patient. Because the lenses will be worn in the normal state, the latent refraction is not of any practical value.

In performing the refraction, give the least amount of cylinder that gives the best-corrected Snellen line. That is, if the patient can just make out the 20/20 line with 1.25 diopters of cylinder but will accept 2.00 diopters of cylinder to read the same line, choose the lower cylinder amount for the contact lens Rx. Small lens rotation will be less noticeable to the patient if the cylinder is smaller.

ANALYZE ASTIGMATISM IN REFRACTION

If the cylinder is between 1 and 2 diopters, use a front toric lens for any of the types of astigmatism; use a back toric lens if the astigmatism is pure corneal.

If the cylinder is 3 diopters or greater and is pure corneal, choose a back toric lens. This is common with patients with high astigmatism. If this is not the case, order a custom front toric lens.

TRIAL LENS

It is worth noting that the *Rx of the lens has been established before placing a trial lens.* The placement of this lens is only to assess comfort, base curve, and stability. Several brands should be at hand. I routinely use a thick/thin-zoned lens, two styles of prism-ballasted lenses, and one truncated prism-ballasted brand.

The patient is asked to comment on comfort only. Vision is not necessarily tested through these trial lenses. The examiner, by choosing a trial lens close in parameter to his order, can assess fit, movement, centration, and how stable or rotated the lens behaves. The best-appearing lens for this patient is chosen, and the base curve and diameter are added to the order.

NO LARS AT THIS STEP

No rotation adjustments are made during this stage of fitting. The lens is ordered and dispensed. If the vision at the time of dispensing is 20/40 or better, the patient is told to build up his or her wearing time and to return in 2 weeks.

FOLLOW-UP

It is at this time that stability and rotations are dealt with. Spherical power can be tested over the lens. Do not try to refract cylinder over the lens. If the lens has rotated, use LARS to reorder a lens. If a creeping or erratic rotation occurs, refit base curve and leave Rx power and axis alone.

Why wait 2 weeks? These delicate adjustments are more reliable on an adapted eye.

Following these steps, 85–90% success should be expected.

FINAL NOTE

Experience, as in all things that are new, will be the greatest teacher with this type of lens. If you have never fit this lens before, start with patients who are sure winners.

1. Choose a patient with astigmatism in one eye only. Fit one eye with a regular soft lens, and fit the other eye with a soft toric lens.
2. Choose a patient with much more spherical error than astigmatic error ($-5.00 - 1.00 \times 90$). There is a better chance for success than in the case of a patient with $-1.00 - 1.00 \times 90$. The astigmatism is more significant in the latter patient.
3. Choose cylinders of 90° and 180°. Avoid oblique axes until you are more experienced.
4. Choose myopes over hyperopes. They are usually better motivated and more easily pleased.

APPENDIX: EXAMPLES OF FITTING

ASTIGMATISM ANALYSIS

1. A 20-year-old patient would like soft lenses and has never worn lenses before:

$$\text{O.U. } F_m: \quad -2.00 + 2.00 \times 90$$

$$\text{O.U. } K: \quad 43/45 \times 90$$

ANALYSIS: Pure corneal astigmatism—Proceed with front or back toric lens.

2. A 30-year-old would like soft lenses and has never worn lenses before:

$$\text{O.U. } F_m: \quad -2.00 + 2.00 \times 180$$

$$\text{O.U. } K_a: \quad 43 \text{ sphere}$$

ANALYSIS: Against-the-rule lenticular astigmatism—Use a front toric lens.

3. An 18-year-old patient wore PMMA lenses briefly, then tried 02 permeable lenses for several months. The patient has been told that he has an astigmatism and can't wear soft lenses.

$$F_m: \quad -2.00 + 2.00 \times 180$$

$$K_a: \quad 43/44 \times 90$$

ANALYSIS: Residual lenticular astigmatism—Use front toric lenses. **Note:** The rigid lenses could only correct the astigmatism that was corneal. The vision will be better with soft toric lenses than with rigid lenses for this reason.

4. A 35-year-old patient has PMMA lens failure. She discontinued lenses because of poor vision and comfort.

$$F_m: \quad -4.00 \text{ sphere}$$

$$K: \quad 43/45 \times 90$$

ANALYSIS: Favorable corneal astigmatism—Use soft spherical lenses.

5. LARS:

$$F_m: \quad -5.00 + 2.00 \times 90$$

$$K: \quad 42/44 \times 90$$

ANALYSIS: Pure corneal astigmatism—Front toric is chosen and ordered as $-3.00 - 200 \times 180$. Lens is worn for 2 weeks. Vision is then 20/40. Lens rotates stably to the examiner's right, 20°. Lens should be reordered as $-3.00 - 2.00 \times 160$. Patient is dispensed a new lens, then vision improved.

6. Same problem as number 4, but now the reordered lens doesn't rotate the same as before. **Solution:** Try a different lens; perhaps a back toric or front toric, with greater stability.

ACKNOWLEDGMENTS

I would like to express my gratitude to the following individuals: Hank Greene, Vistakon, Inc., for his assistance with graphics and photos; Barry Maltzman, M.D., for his assistance with graphics; and Maureen McDonald, for her assistance in typing and preparing the manuscript for this chapter.

BIBLIOGRAPHY

1. Baglien, J. W. The use of toric corneal contact lenses. *Optom. Weekly*, 44:129, 1953.

2. Bailey, N. J. Contact lens update, part 2. *Contact Lens Forum*, 7:29, 1982.

3. Bayshore, C. A. Astigmatis soft contact lenses: A report on 88 patients. *Int. Contact Lens Clin.*, 2:68, 1975.

4. Bayshore, C. A. Soft toric lenses we can live with. *Contact Lens*, 7:29, 1982.

5. Brummel, A. J. Fenestrations to fight lens rotation. *Contact Lens Forum*, 6:17, 1981.

6. Callendar, M. G. E., and Egan, D. A clinical evaluation on the Weicon-T and Durasoft TT soft contact lenses. *Int. Contact Lens Clin.*, 5:209, 1978.

7. Dain, S. J. Overrefraction and axis mislocation of toric lenses. *Int. Contact Lens Clin.*, 6:57, 1979.

8. Ewell, D. G. Clinical application of toric soft lenses. *Contact Lens Forum*, 5:23, 1980.

9. Fink, B. A., and Tomlinson, A. A comparison of three methods of measurement of toric soft lens orientation. *Am. J. Optom. Physiol. Opt.*, 59:611, 1982.

10. Gasson, A. The correction of astigmatism and Hydroflex toric soft lenses. *Contact Lens J.*, 8:3, 1979.

11. Hallak, J. Standard soft toric lenses: A problem of orientation. *Int. Contact Lens Clin.*, 9:250, 1982.

12. Hirst, G. Recent developments in hard and hydrophilic aspheric contact lenses, and the use of toric and bifocal hydrophilic lenses. *Contacto*, 24:35, 1980.

13. Burnett Hodd, N. F. How to fit soft lenses-10, Toric soft lenses (part 2). *Optician*, 173:8, 1977.

14. Holden, G. A. The principles and practice of correcting astigmatism with soft contact lenses. *Aust. J. Optom.*, 58:279, 1975.

15. Hott, W. Soft toric contact lenses. *Optician*, 175:29, 1978.

16. Jurkus, J. M., and Tomlinson, A. Prism-ballasted and truncated spherical trial lenses as indicators of toric soft lens rotation. *Am. J. Optom. Physiol. Opt.*, 56:16, 1979.

17. Jurkus, J., Tomlinson, A., Bilbault, D. C., et al. The effect of fit and parameter changes on soft lens rotation. *Am. J. Optom. Physiol. Opt.*, 56:734, 1979.

18. Korb, D. R. A preliminary report on toric contact lenses. *Optom. Weekly*, 51:2501, 1960.

19. Korb, D. R. A preliminary report of continuing performance of toric inner surface contact lenses. *Contacto*, 5:317, 1961.

20. Kress, J. A. Results of experiments with new hydrogel toric lenses. *Int. Contact Lens Clin.*, 4:64, 1977.

21. Leiblein, J. S. A study of the Durasoft toric contact lens for astigmatism, and a fitting rationale. *Int. Contact Lens Clin.*, 7:21, 1980.

22. Malin, A. H., and Kohler, J. Measuring toric rotation. *Contact Lens Forum*, 6:17, 1981.

23. Maltzman, B. A., Fruchman, D., Nostrame, S., et al. Axis stability and toric soft lenses. *Contact Intraocul. Lens Med. J.*, 17:53, 1981.

24. Maltzman, B. A., Koeniger, E., and Dabenzies, O. H. In: Dabenzies, O. H. (Ed.), *Contact Lens: The CLAO Guide to Basic Science Clinical Practice*, Chapter 51, pp. 51.1–51.15, Grune & Stratton, New York, 1984.

25. Maltzman, B. A., and Parariello A: Toric soft lenses. Contact Intraocul. Lens Med. J., 5:168, 1979.

26. Mandel, R. B. *Contact Lens Practice: Basic and Advanced.* Charles C. Thomas, Springfield, Illinois, 1965.

27. Muckenhirn, D. Weiche tori-linsen in Neuer Konzeption. *Neuesoptiker J.*, 144, 1973.

28. Peet, C. The Weicon toric—the manufacturers' and practitioners' views. *Optician*, 177:22, 1979.

29. Raskin, N. Fitting Hydron toric lenses. *Contact Lens Forum*, 7:103, 1982.

30. Remba, J. M. Part II: Clinical evaluation of toric hydrophilic contact lenses. *J. Am. Optom. Assoc.*, 52:211, 1981.

31. Remba, J. M. Clinical efficacy of toric soft lenses. *Int. Contact Lens Clin.*, 8:26, 1981.

32. Remba, M. J. The ABC's of toric lens fitting. *Rev. Optom.*, 99:25, 1962.

33. Ruben, M. *Contact Lens Practice: Visual, Therapeutic and Prosthetic.* Williams and Wilkins, Baltimore, 1975.

34. Salvatori, A. L. Bal-flange toric: A new contact lens for non-rational orientation. *Int. Contact Lens Clin.*, 9:355, 1982.

35. Shapiro, M. A review of a new corneal contact lens. *Optom. Weekly*, 43:713, 1952.

36. Shapiro, M. The fitting of highly toric corneas with toric corneal contact lenses. *Am. J. Optom.*, 30:157, 1953.

37. Soni, P. S., Borish, I. M., and Keech, P. M., Corneal thickness changes with toric soft lenses: Prism-ballasted versus nonprism-ballasted design. *Int. Contact Lens Clin.*, 6:196, 1979.

38. Soni, P. S., and Tomlinson, A. Astigmatic correction with Durasoft TT contact lenses. *Rev. Optom.*, 116:63, 1979.

39. Tomlinson, A., Schoessier, J. and Andrasko, G. The effect of varying prism and truncation on the performance of soft contact lenses. *Am. J. Optom. Physiol. Opt.*, 57:714, 1980.

40. Wesley, N. K. A new contact lens for toroidal eyes. *Opt. J. Rev. Optom.*, 97:39, 1960.

6
BIFOCAL AND MULTIFOCAL CONTACT LENSES

FRANK J. WEINSTOCK, M.D., F.A.C.S.

INDICATIONS

Multifocal contact lenses are indicated (Table 6.1) for the motivated contact lens candidate who has the need for distant and near refractive correction (Fig. 6.1). This candidate is primarily the presbyopic patient who can no longer perform near visual tasks with his or her single-vision lenses (Figs. 6.2 and 6.3). By experience it has been shown that the individual who does not require glasses continually for distance will not tolerate a bifocal contact lens. If these individuals desire contact lenses, they are candidates for the monovision technique, which will be discussed below.

Since most cataract surgery is now performed with the use of intraocular lens implants, multifocal contact lenses have a limited use after cataract surgery (Figs. 6.4 and 6.5). However, patients who no longer wish to wear spectacles may be excellent candidates for multifocal contact lenses. This may help to im-

TABLE 6.1 INDICATIONS
Presbyopia with significant distant refraction— new contact lens patient
Previous single-vision wearer
Motivated patient
Cosmetic
Occupational needs
Postoperative cataract surgery—without implant —with implant
Accommodative esotropia

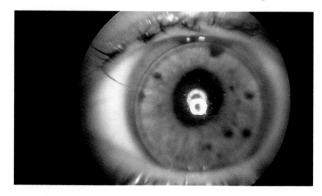

Fig. 6.1 *Aphakic eye of patient who has successfully worn hard, crescent segmented bifocal lenses for 15 years.*

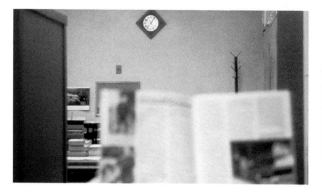

Fig. 6.2 *Presbyopia—without correction.*

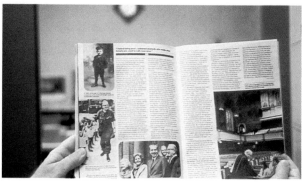

Fig. 6.3 *Presbyopia—with correction.*

prove the outlook of a patient who may have been depressed over the presence of a cataract and the need for surgery.

Another type of patient who may do well with multifocal contact lenses is the patient with accommodative esotropia. The simultaneous vision (see below) concept is particularly successful in this situation (Figs. 6.6 and 6.7).

Occasionally, patients do not require lenses for distant vision and only want contacts for intermittent wear such as public appearances, going out to restaurants, etc.

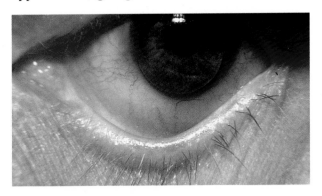

Fig. 6.4 *Phakic eye—Boston IV executive bifocal.*

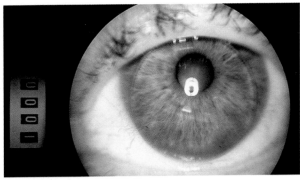

Fig. 6.5 *Aphakic fellow eye with implant and Boston IV executive bifocal.*

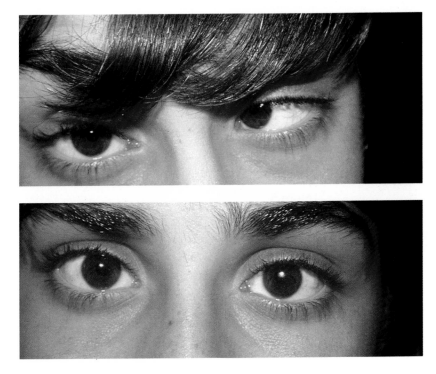

Fig. 6.6 *Accommodative esotropia—without bifocal contact lens.*

Fig. 6.7 *Accommodative esotropia—corrected with VFL aspheric bifocal lens.*

CONTRAINDICATIONS

The contraindications (Table 6.2) for multifocal contact lenses are the same as for single-vision lenses, with some additions. Lenses should not be considered for use in patients with chronic conjunctivitis, blepharitis, or keratitis, in patients who have poor hygiene, in patients who cannot handle contact lenses (e.g., those with severe arthritis), or in patients who are unreliable and cannot follow instructions or take adequate care of lenses. Patients with no significant distant refractive error, patients with narrow palpebral fissures (not an absolute contraindication), and patients with poor motivation should not be fit.

Depending upon the ability of the specific lens to provide adequate near correction, it may be necessary to avoid certain lenses when the near vision tasks are demanding. Certain lens types and materials provide minimal "add power" and require significant compromises by the patient.

TABLE 6.2
CONTRAINDICATIONS

Poor motivation
Chronic conjunctivitis and/or blepharitis
Poor hygiene
No significant distant refraction
Narrow palpebral fissures (in many patients)

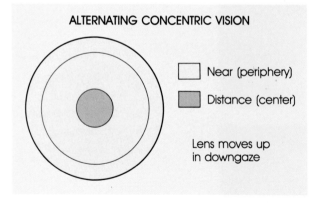

Fig. 6.8 *Alternating-vision concentric bifocal lens.*

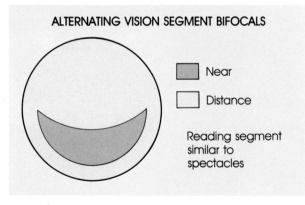

Fig. 6.9 *Alternating-vision segmented bifocal lens.*

THEORY AND MATERIALS

Multifocal contact lenses function by one of two mechanisms:

1. Alternating vision.
   a. Segmented design.
   b. Concentric or annular design.
2. Simultaneous vision.
   a. Aspheric design.
   b. Concentric or annular design.

These mechanisms also form the basis for the use of a combination of a single-vision lens and a bifocal lens for the modified monovision technique.

ALTERNATING VISION

Alternating-vision contact lenses (Figs. 6.8–6.11) ("dual-purpose" lenses) are similar to standard segmented bifocal spectacles, having one portion (usually the upper or central portion of the lens) for distant viewing and one portion (usually the lower or

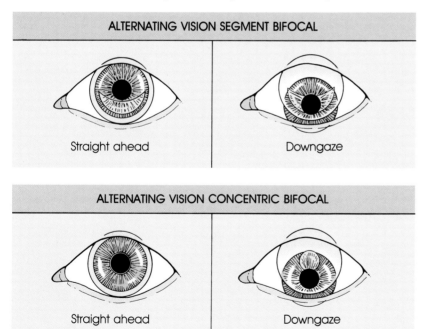

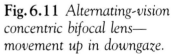
Fig. 6.10 *Alternating-vision segmented bifocal lens— movement up in downgaze.*

Fig. 6.11 *Alternating-vision concentric bifocal lens— movement up in downgaze.*

peripheral portion of the lens) for near viewing (Fig. 6.12). In these lenses the patient views distant objects through the top or central portion of the lens. For viewing near objects, the patient looks down and the lens is shifted up to allow a clear view through the lower or peripheral portion of the lens. The eye and the brain will concentrate on one clear image at a time (either the distant or the near image) (Figs. 6.13 and 6.14; Table 6.3).

Fig. 6.12 *Crescent segmented alternating-vision bifocal contact lens.*

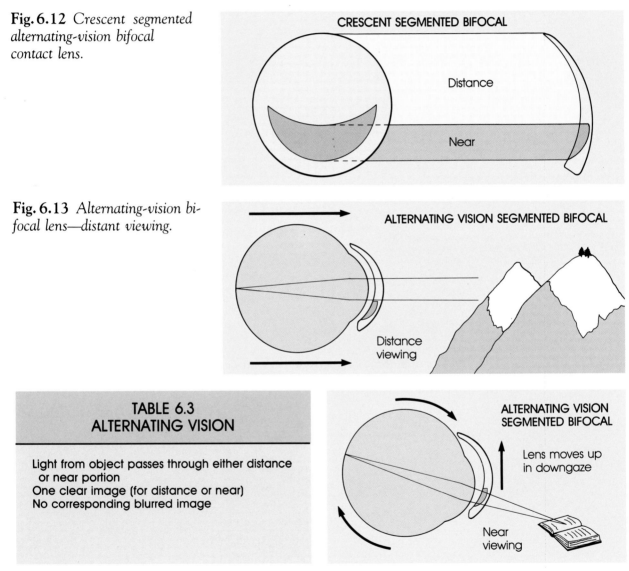

CRESCENT SEGMENTED BIFOCAL

Distance

Near

Fig. 6.13 *Alternating-vision bifocal lens—distant viewing.*

ALTERNATING VISION SEGMENTED BIFOCAL

Distance viewing

TABLE 6.3
ALTERNATING VISION

Light from object passes through either distance or near portion
One clear image (for distance or near)
No corresponding blurred image

ALTERNATING VISION SEGMENTED BIFOCAL

Lens moves up in downgaze

Near viewing

Fig. 6.14 *Alternating-vision bifocal lens—near viewing.*

BIFOCAL AND MULTIFOCAL CONTACT LENSES

SIMULTANEOUS VISION

Simultaneous-vision lenses ("selective-vision" lenses) usually do not have a specific near segment (except for the Alges bifocal with the central near portion and the peripheral distant portion). They may be annular or aspheric and work on the principle that multiple images for near and distant objects are projected on the retina (Figs. 6.15 and 6.16). The individual selectively concentrates on the desired image and suppresses the other images. When an individual looks at a distant object the distant rays form a clear image on the macula, with the near rays forming a blurred diffusion circle on the macula. For a near object the near rays will form the clear image on the macula, with the distant rays forming the blurred diffusion circle. The individual learns to concentrate on the clear image and to ignore the blurred image (Tables 6.4–6.6). Since all rays passing through the lens

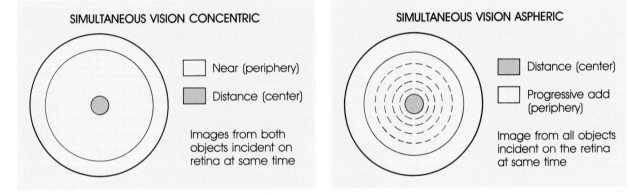

Fig. 6.15 *Simultaneous-vision concentric bifocal lens.*

Fig. 6.16 *Simultaneous-vision aspheric bifocal lens.*

TABLE 6.4 SIMULTANEOUS VISION	TABLE 6.5 SIMULTANEOUS VISION— DISTANCE VIEWING	TABLE 6.6 SIMULTANEOUS VISION— NEAR VIEWING
Light rays from object viewed simultaneously pass through distant and near portion of lens Concentrate on clear image Ignore blurred image	Distant portion of rays focus on macula Near portion of rays focus in front of retina (blurred diffusion circle; shadow around objects) Concentrate on distant rays Ignore near (blurred) rays	Near portion of rays focus on macula Distant portion of rays focus behind retina (blurred diffusion circle) Concentrate on near rays Ignore distance rays

must be focused in the macular region at all times, it is essential that these lenses be relatively stable on the cornea, with minimal movement. Another type of simultaneous vision is provided by a lens with the near segment in the center and the distance correction in the periphery of the lens.

Besides the fact that many individuals find it difficult, if not impossible, to "learn" to use simultaneous-vision lenses, the near vision effect is often less than desired. It is rarely possible to achieve the higher adds that are obtained with alternating-vision lenses. Because of this, it is frequently necessary to compromise between distant and near vision.

MONOVISION

Although this method usually does not incorporate a multifocal lens, it is frequently used for individuals who have need for a presbyopic correction. Erroneously, it is often referred to as "bi-focal" fitting. Standard single-vision lenses are used to correct one eye for distance and one eye for near viewing.

MODIFIED MONOVISION

A standard single-vision lens is used for the distant correction on one eye, with a multifocal lens on the other eye for near viewing. This usually is a simultaneous-vision lens which, theoretically, will provide a wider range of near vision than a segmented bifocal. It occasionally works well as a true multifocal lens, thus affording binocular distant vision and monocular near vision.

When considering monovision or modified monovision fitting, some patients voice a concern about the possible loss of binocularity and the potential interference with depth perception. No major studies have been undertaken to prove or disprove this consideration. There have been some small studies that indicate no significant interference with binocularity. In addition, discussion with happy monovision patients indicates that they have no problems with depth perception, driving, reading, etc. On the other hand, there are some patients who feel extremely unbalanced and feel that they are unable to tolerate monovision fitting.

MATERIALS

ALTERNATING-VISION LENSES

DAILY-WEAR LENSES Multifocal lenses are available in soft or rigid materials. The rigid lenses are available in either polymethylmethacrylate (PMMA) or gas-permeable materials.

The alternating-vision principle requires a lens that is able to translate by moving up on the eye to allow clear vision through the bifocal. In addition, the near portion of the lens must have a different refractive power than the distant portion. This usually requires that the near segment or peripheral annular segment be thicker than the distant portion.

POLYMETHYLMETHACRYLATE (PMMA) HARD LENSES
The manufacturing of PMMA bifocal lenses usually involves fusing two plastics with different indices of refraction. This will produce a lens which may function perfectly, but which is thicker and heavier than a single-vision lens. This type of bifocal lens is commonly referred to as a *segmented lens* or *crescent segmented lens*, with the near-vision segment appearing as a half-moon configuration (Fig. 6.17). This configuration is modified by individual companies. Some individuals will not be able to tolerate these characteristics and will have discomfort or may incur corneal hypoxia (probably due to the greater mass of the lens), with resulting intolerance of the lens.

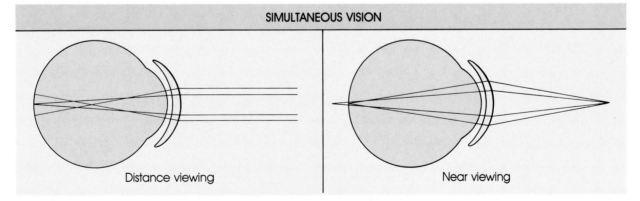

Fig. 6.17 *Simultaneous vision—distant and near viewing.*

RIGID GAS-PERMEABLE LENSES (RGP OR GPL) With gas-permeable lenses, it is technically difficult to fuse another plastic to the original lens. Instead, masking the distant portion and grinding the lens to incorporate the bifocal near addition in the inferior portion of the lens will produce a bifocal lens which is referred to as an *executive bifocal.*

As opposed to the fusing process used in the hard lenses whereby the separation of the two segments is abrupt and sharp, it is currently technically difficult to achieve a perfectly sharp demarcation line between the distant and near vision. This may result in some glare or flare.

These lenses are heavier and thicker than conventional single-vision lenses, thus making them somewhat more difficult to fit and to wear. If the lens moves too much, there will be unsteady, poor translation between sharp distant and near vision. In spite of excellent optics, some patients do not attain sufficiently sharp vision.

Occasionally, the alternating-vision lenses of either PMMA, soft, or gas-permeable material may be ground as an annular bifocal lens, with the central portion of the lens providing distant vision and the peripheral annular portion being used for near vision. Although this should function as well as the crescent segmented or executive bifocal, it often is not as effective in general.

SOFT HYDROGEL LENSES There are major technical problems in producing an effective soft alternating-vision bifocal. These lenses must be thicker than the standard soft lens and should move up in order to look through the bifocal. Comfort and good vision for distance and near viewing are rarely attained with the soft alternating-vision bifocals. Efforts are continually directed toward finding a satisfactory soft bifocal lens. Each company has its own material and design with specific parameters and fitting characteristics.

SIMULTANEOUS-VISION LENSES
Simultaneous-vision lenses are easier to manufacture and are available in hard, gas-permeable, or soft materials.

EXTENDED-WEAR LENSES Extended-wear lenses are available in gas-permeable or soft materials. Although many lenses are being evaluated for extended-wear capabilities, relatively few have been approved for use. At the time of this writing, there are no bifocal or multifocal contact lenses approved for extended wear.

However, extended-wear lenses of either gas-permeable or soft materials function extremely well for patients who wish to use the monovision method for presbyopic correction.

FITTING

Fitting of multifocal and bifocal contact lenses is individualized for each lens type, company, and material. Each company will have a "cookbook" to be followed for indications, fitting, and results. Alternating-vision lenses are fit by use of principles that are similar to those used for single-vision lenses. However, simultaneous-vision or aspheric lenses are usually fit in a completely different fashion.

In addition, a fitting set (Fig. 6.18) is recommended for attaining the best possible success. Each lens type and each company will have a specific fitting set for the lens to be used. This is cumbersome and expensive. Familiarity with the available lenses and their success rates will enable the practitioner to decide which lenses should be used.

Depending upon the lens to be used, the manufacturing parameters of specific lenses may limit the choice of patients. For example, some lenses may not provide good vision in patients with astigmatism or in patients who require high adds or high plus or minus corrections.

HOW TO FIT

Because multifocal and bifocal contact lenses have specific characteristics in reference to how to fit and how the lens sits and functions on the eye, it is desirable to utilize a diagnostic fitting set of lenses in the fitting procedure. The diagnostic set of lenses

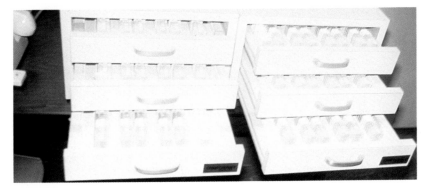

Fig. 6.18 *Diagnostic fitting set.*

allows one to evaluate the fit from the standpoint of size, base curve, and location of the segment (where applicable) and to over-refract in order to obtain the best near and distant vision.

Each lens is different from the standpoint of material, mode of action, and company characteristics, thereby making it necessary to have a different set of lenses for each lens type utilized. Obviously this can be very expensive. Most practitioners will concentrate on a small number of types of lenses and have fitting sets for these lenses. A fitting guide ("cookbook") is usually required for each lens type. Because of this, the guidelines for fitting that follow (Table 6.7) may not pertain to some lenses.

DAILY-WEAR LENSES

These may be monovision, alternating-vision, or simultaneous-vision designs. There are many alternatives available, depending upon the patient's previous contact lens experience and needs as well as the contemplated uses of the lenses.

CHOICES FOR THE PATIENT REQUIRING NEAR CORRECTION
A patient may wear bifocal glasses without contact lenses, may wear contact lenses with bifocal or reading glasses over the contacts, may use the monovision or modified monovision technique, or may wear bifocal contact lenses.

The easiest method is to avoid bifocal lenses and use the monovision method, which may be quite successful. If the patient is an early presbyope and has been wearing single-vision lenses successfully, it is often simplest to decrease the minus in the nondominant eye and continue with single-vision lenses. This requires a minimal amount of adaptation on the part of the patient. It is also much more economical.

Preferably the new patient is fit with an alternating bifocal contact lens in gas-permeable or PMMA material. If the patient

---

TABLE 6.7
FITTING MULTIFOCAL LENSES

Keratometry
Refraction
Diagnostic lens (initial lens size and base curve from individual company fitting guide)
Evaluate fit (base curve, size, segment) where applicable
Over-refract
Order lens

specifically desires a soft lens, either a multifocal simultaneous vision lens or a modified monovision method of fitting is used.

MONOVISION TECHNIQUE With the individual who has been a successful single-vision contact lens wearer, plus power may be added to the nondominant eye for reading (Table 6.8). If this is begun at the onset of presbyopia, the chance of acceptance by the patient is better. The small amount of plus may only reduce the distance vision by one to two lines and may not be very noticeable. This also allows the patient to continue with single-vision lenses with which he or she is familiar.

A simple method of determining the eye to be used for reading is to use the opposite eye to the dominant hand. With right-handed patients, the nondominant left eye is usually used for reading; with left-handed patients, the right eye is usually used. Or you may ask the patient to look through a pinhole, finding that the patient uses the dominant eye to look through the pinhole with the opposite eye being used for near vision.

The fitting method for monovision is the same as for any single-vision lenses and will follow that of hard, soft, or gas-permeable single-vision lenses on a daily- or extended-wear basis (Figs. 6.19 and 6.20). The reading lens is placed upon one eye,

TABLE 6.8 MONOVISION TECHNIQUE	
Successful single-vision patient	Distant lens on dominant eye
Unsuccessful multifocal patient	Near lens on nondominant eye
Single-vison lenses	

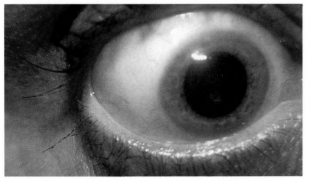

Fig. 6.19 *Monovision—Cooper extended-wear soft lens on left eye for distant viewing.*

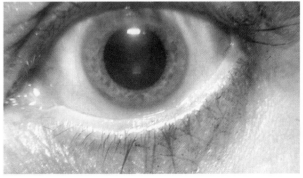

Fig. 6.20 *Monovision—Cooper extended-wear soft lens on right eye for near viewing.*

or the plus can be placed in a trial frame for the patient to try in the office. If the patient isn't happy, the lenses can be switched and the reading can be tried with the other eye. As with all near-vision lenses, it is desired to keep the plus as low as possible.

The *modified* monovision technique (Table 6.9) involves a single-vision lens for distant vision and a simultaneous-vision multifocal lens on the other eye for near vision. Theoretically, in addition to the near vision, better intermediate vision is provided. The fitting procedure for the near eye will follow the routine for the specific simultaneous-vision lens to be used. In general a soft lens will be used.

Some patients cannot or will not accept the monovision or modified monovision technique because of a sense of imbalance caused by the difference between the two eyes. If the only complaint is for distant vision, a third single-vision lens for distance may be used when near vision is not required, or spectacles that neutralize the near-vision lens may be used while driving, etc.

Bifocal contact lenses should be used if the above alternatives are not successful. I prefer to fit multifocal or bifocal contact lenses over monovision whenever possible. An exception may be the early presbyope who has been wearing single-vision contact lenses successfully, especially if the lenses are soft.

FITTING MULTIFOCAL OR BIFOCAL CONTACT LENSES
Although some guidelines for fitting will be given, each company has a specific fitting procedure for each lens, whether hard, soft, or gas-permeable.

I do not feel that it is necessary to carry out a pre-bifocal fitting with a single-vision lens. If a patient desires to be fit with bifocal lenses, it is done primarily directly at the time of the exam. It only takes a few minutes longer than fitting single-

---

TABLE 6.9
MODIFIED MONOVISION TECHNIQUE

Distant single-vision lens on dominant eye
Multifocal simultaneous-vision lens on
nondominant eye

TABLE 6.10
FITTING PREVIOUS SINGLE-VISION HARD LENS PATIENT
(With Segmented Hard Lens)

Same base curve as successful single-vision lens
Increase diameter by 0.2 mm
Increase optical zone by 0.2 mm
Segment height should be 0.1 mm below
  optical zone, or use diagnostic lens
Same near add as for glasses

vision lenses. It is rarely necessary to use topical anesthetic drops, except for cases where the patient is tearing excessively.

If a patient has been wearing hard single-vision lenses successfully and wishes to continue with hard lenses (Table 6.10), a segmented hard lens may be ordered, with the only modification being the addition of 0.2 mm to the overall diameter (this also adds 0.2 mm to the size of the optical zone) of the lens. Although this may be accomplished without the use of a fitting set, it is still desirable to use a fitting set prior to ordering the final lens and to observe the lens on the eye.

HARD DAILY-WEAR CONTACT LENSES (PMMA)

SEGMENTED LENSES (TABLE 6.11) Because these lenses have a spherical posterior surface, they are fit using the same principles as used for a single-vision lens, utilizing the single-vision formula for choosing the initial base curve of the diagnostic lens. This is usually 0.25–0.5 diopter steeper than the flattest K, with modifications according to the amount of astigmatism. Choose a lens that corresponds to one-third the difference between the K readings.

The lens is usually 9.0–9.2 mm in size, with the height of the segment being on the geometric center (G.C.) or 0.1 or 0.2 mm below the G.C. With high minus prescriptions it may be lower (0.3 mm below the G.C.), and with aphakes or patients with small pupils it may be higher (on the G.C.).

Alternatively, the segment height may be determined by having the patient look straight ahead and measuring the distance between the edge of the lower lid and the center of the pupil, usually being 4.1–4.3 mm. It is usually better to order a lens with a higher segment than necessary than one that is too low, since it is possible to modify a lens to lower the segment.

TABLE 6.11
HARD CRESCENT SEGMENTED LENSES

Diagnostic lens	Segment: On G.C. or 0.1 mm below G.C.
Initial lens	(lower with high minus and higher with high plus)
Base curve: 0.25–0.50 diopter steeper than	Optical zone: 7.6 mm
flattest K (with significant astigmatism use	Prism ballast: 1.5 diopters down and in
one-third the difference between flat and	Truncation: None
steep K)	Evaluate fit
Size: 9.0–9.2 mm	Over-refract

The optical zone is usually 7.6 mm. If it is modified, it is usually increased.

Prism ballast is used to keep the segment in the proper position. It is usually 1.5 prism diopters down and 10° in.

The peripheral curves would correspond to the normal curves for the size of lens ordered.

Truncation (Fig. 6.21) refers to tapering of the lower edge of the lens for better centration. This is rarely necessary, although some fitters prefer to truncate all lenses routinely.

For greater accuracy a diagnostic fitting set has lenses of varying base curves with prism incorporated, and a horizontal line through the center of the lens is used. The fitting set is used to evaluate the parameters mentioned above; it is also used for over-refraction for distant and near vision. Usually the add will correspond to the add in the spectacle lenses. These lenses are available in virtually all powers and can correct corneal astigmatism.

If a fitting set is not used, it is possible to order a lens based on the keratometry, refraction, and description of the lower lid in relation to the limbus. Avoid fitting patients with narrow palpebral fissures, since they do not adapt well to these lenses.

When the lens is delivered, the teaching and wearing routine is the same as a single-vision lens (Fig. 6.22). It is not necessary to concern oneself with the location of the segment upon inserting, since the prism ballast will automatically orient the lens correctly.

Follow-up (Table 6.12) is also the same as with other hard lenses; it involves checking a patient at intervals—usually a week later and then 2 or 4 weeks later. During the follow-up exams,

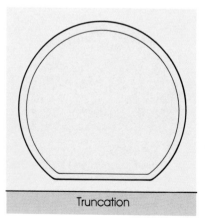

Truncation

Fig. 6.21 *Truncation.*

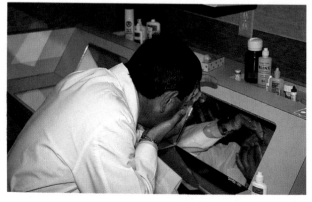

Fig. 6.22 *Photograph of the author, inserting an executive bifocal Boston IV lens.*

BIFOCAL AND MULTIFOCAL CONTACT LENSES

which are made toward the end of the day in the office, the following are checked (this applies to all types of lenses):

1. History—comfort, satisfaction, redness, vision performance.
2. Vision in each eye—distant and near.
3. Over-refraction if necessary.
4. Slit-lamp evaluation of lenses.
5. Slit-lamp evaluation of eye.
6. Observation of fluorescein pattern.
7. Removal of lenses, followed immediately by keratometry and spectacle refraction.

The desired goal is comfortable 20/20 distant vision and 0.37 near vision in each eye, with smooth translation (switching from distant to near vision and the reverse).

PROBLEM SOLVING If a lens is too tight, it may be loosened or blended in the office. If the segment is too high, it may be lowered by flattening the bottom of the lens (truncation). If the segment is too low, a new lens must be ordered.

If the power is not correct, it may be modified in the office, or a new lens may be ordered. Blending might be necessary if the lens is not comfortable. As with spectacles, avoid making the bifocal too strong, since this would require holding objects too close.

If the lens casters (rotates), it may be necessary to order a new lens, specifying the amount of prism desired. Table 6.13 summarizes frequently encountered problems and their solutions.

TABLE 6.12 FOLLOW-UP EXAMS FOR ALL LENSES (Toward the End of the Day)	TABLE 6.13 PROBLEM SOLVING
History—comfort, satisfaction, etc. Vision in each eye—distant and near Over-refraction if necessary Slit-lamp evaluation of lenses—with fluorescein Slit-lamp evaluation of eye—with fluorescein Removal of lenses: Spectacle refraction (should correspond to prefitting) Keratometry (should correspond to prefitting) Slit-lamp evaluation	Uncomfortable: Blend curves Too tight: Loosen Too flat: Order new lens Too much plus: Modify in office Not enough plus or add: Order new lens Segment too high: Flatten or truncate Segment too low: Order new lens Rotation of lens: Order new lens or truncate

SIMULTANEOUS-VISION HARD LENSES

Front aspheric design lenses are fit in a manner similar to any single-vision spherical lens, whereas posterior aspheric lenses are fit 3.0–4.0 diopters steeper, starting with about an 8.7-mm-diameter lens. The base curve and diameter are modified in order to get a lens that centers well on slit-lamp evaluation. Over-refraction is used to arrive at the lens with the least minus necessary to provide good vision.

Aspheric lenses are dispensed in the same manner as any hard lens, but it is often necessary to arrive at a visual compromise whereby distant and near vision may be somewhat less than perfect. It appears that many "successful" patients end up with a modified monovision situation, using one eye for distant vision and one eye for near vision.

GAS-PERMEABLE DAILY-WEAR LENSES

EXECUTIVE BIFOCAL (ROONEY) An example of an alternating-vision gas-permeable lens is the Rooney executive bifocal (Rooney Optical Company, Cleveland, Ohio), which is fit from a diagnostic set of lenses with concentric circles for determining the segment height and prism to determine rotation (Table 6.14 and Figs. 6.23 and 6.24). The base curve is chosen in the same manner as would be done with a single-vision lens, usually 0.25 diopter steeper than the flattest K. The most common size is 9.5 mm, with the goal being a well-centering lens with slight movement and good translation in downgaze for reading. Over-refraction is carried out for each eye for distant and near vision, aiming for 20/20 distant vision and 0.37-m near vision, avoiding making the bifocal too strong. There are no power restrictions, and significant corneal astigmatism may be masked.

The location of the dot on the diagnostic lens is noted by clock hour for use by the lab in correctly locating the prism for proper orientation of the bifocal.

TABLE 6.14
GAS-PERMEABLE EXECUTIVE BIFOCAL LENSES

Base curve: 0.25 diopter steeper than flattest K
Size: 9.5 mm
Segment height: Choose concentric ring (at lower edge of pupil)
Evaluate fit
Give lab power of spectacle refraction
Order lens

BIFOCAL AND MULTIFOCAL CONTACT LENSES

Four concentric rings, 1 mm apart, are cut on the front surface of the lens for location of the bifocal segment (Fig. 6.25). This should be at the lower edge of the pupil in dim light. Measurement under the colored beam of the slit lamp may be a little more reliable than the brighter illumination. Although the central circle is 1.2 mm below the geometric center of the lens, the segment height is ordered by mentioning the circle desired. Since the concentric circles for determining the segment height might interfere with an over-refraction, the laboratory will determine the correct peripheral curves and the power from the spectacle refraction.

Dispense the lenses as you would dispense any other GPL, with the same care and fitting regimen as a single-vision lens and with a goal of excellent distant and near vision, recognizing that there may be some extra glare, especially at night.

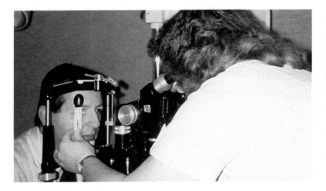

Fig. 6.23 *Slit-lamp evaluation—checking bifocal segment height with a millimeter rule.*

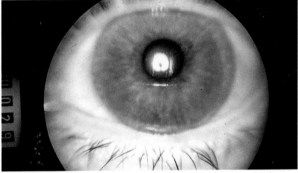

Fig. 6.24 *Boston IV executive bifocal (Rooney Optical Company, Cleveland, Ohio).*

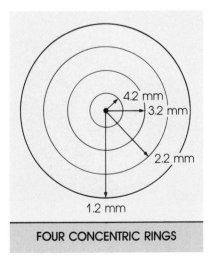

FOUR CONCENTRIC RINGS

4.2 mm
3.2 mm
2.2 mm
1.2 mm

Fig. 6.25 *Circles on diagnostic lens—used for determining segment height.*

BIFOCAL AND MULTIFOCAL CONTACT LENSES

TANGENT STREAK BIFOCALS (FUSED KONTACTS)

The Tangent Streak gas-permeable bifocal contact lens from Fused Kontacts (Chicago, Illinois) is fit from a 20-lens fitting set (Fig. 6.26). It is available in lens sizes of 8.00–10.50 mm, base curves of 6.50–8.50 mm, distance powers from +20.00 to −20.00 diopters and adds of +0.75–2.00 diopters.

This truncated lens, which is fit flat, positions low in primary position and translates upward in reading position. (Figs. 6.27, 6.28, 6.29.) With a spherical cornea it is fit 1.00 diopter flatter than "K," with no lens being fit any steeper than one fourth of the toricity when astigmatism is over 1.00 diopter. Prism, with truncation, orients the lens low in order for the lower lid to displace the lens upward for near viewing.

Over-refraction determines the power, whereas the size and segment height are related to the position of the lower lid in reference to the lower edge of the lens and the visual axis. These measurements are taken with a ruler (or reticule in the slit lamp) while the patient looks at a penlight held at eye level at a distance of about 20 inches. 1.3 mm is subtracted from the lower lid to the visual axis for the segment height. If the lid is flush with or higher than the lower limbus, the segment height is determined by subtracting 1.3 mm from the measured distance (in millimeters) between the lower lid margin and the visual axis (center of the cornea). If the lid is below the lower limbus, a larger lens with a higher segment and larger truncation is used. This lens does not perform well and is contraindicated if the lower lid is flaccid or 1.5 mm or more below the limbus.

The ophthalmologist dispenses these lenses, and the wearer adapts to them, in much the same way as in the case of other

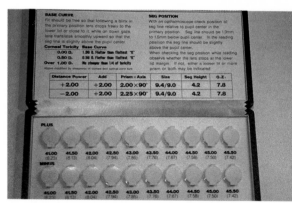

Fig. 6.26 *Diagnostic fitting set.*

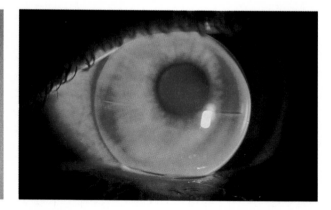

Fig. 6.27 *Proper positioning.*

gas-permeable lenses, except that there may be increased flare due to the segment.

Recently the Alges bifocal (see details in subsection on soft lenses) has become available in gas-permeable materials. The details of fitting are not available at this time, but best results probably will be obtained from a fitting set, aiming for a well-centering lens.

PROBLEM SOLVING (EXECUTIVE BIFOCAL OR TANGENT STREAK) The most common problem (Table 6.15) is that of segment height, which might require truncation or reordering the lens. Power corrections might also require new lenses. Glare complaints must be understood by the patient and might not be correctable. Poor truncation may require a looser lens, modification of truncation, or a lower segment. A lens that is too tight translates poorly, yields poor reading vision, and must

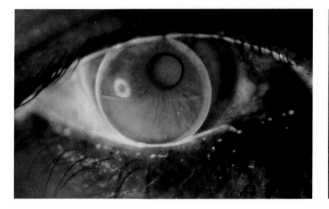

Fig. 6.28 *Proper alignment.*

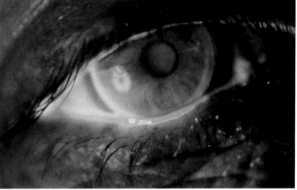

Fig. 6.29 *Correct upward displacement in reading position.*

TABLE 6.15 PROBLEM SOLVING
Power correction: Order new lens Incorrect bifocal height: Order new lens Too much glare: Order new lens (stressing polishing)

be made looser (Fig. 6.30). A lens which is too loose will decenter temporally (Fig. 6.31).

HARD OR GAS-PERMEABLE OR SIMULTANEOUS-VISION POSTERIOR ASPHERIC LENSES

An example is the APA aspheric lens of GBF contact lenses (Table 6.16).

A table is used to determine the base curve which is 4.00–5.50 diopters steeper than the flattest K, or a diagnostic lens 4.00 diopters steeper may be chosen for the initial lens. This lens is then evaluated for fit, seeking a well-fitting alignment with a uniform-depth edge-to-edge dye pattern under the lens which centers well (Fig. 6.32).

A lens is too steep (Fig. 6.33) if the central dye pattern is deep with an apical bubble and with poor movement of blinking.

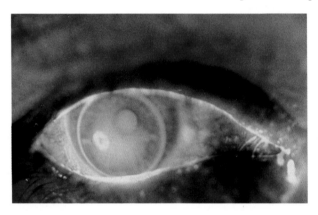

Fig. 6.30 *Too steep; lens will not displace up for reading position.*

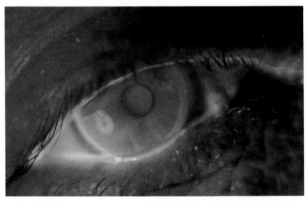

Fig. 6.31 *Flat lens decenters temporally.*

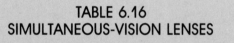

TABLE 6.16
SIMULTANEOUS-VISION LENSES

Diagnostic lens: Choose according to guidebook
Base curve: 3–5.50 diopters steeper than
  flattest K
Size: 8.7 mm
Evaluate fit
Over-refract distant and near vision using
  trial frame
Order lens

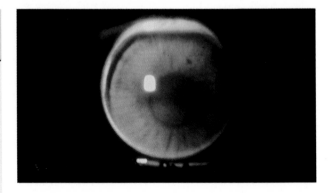

Fig. 6.32 *Well-fitting rigid aspheric bifocal.*

BIFOCAL AND MULTIFOCAL CONTACT LENSES

There may be peripheral touch also with fluorescein (Fig. 6.34). In contrast, a loose lens will have (a) a diffuse fluorescein dye pattern with apical bearing and (b) an absence of dye centrally with excessive lens movement.

To arrive at the proper base curve, lenses are fit progressively steeper by increasing the radii in 0.1-mm increments until a bubble forms in the apical area. The next flatter lens is then chosen with the fluorescein pattern, while centration and lens movement is being observed. The lens should center well with no more than 1.5–2 mm of decentration in the primary position and no more than 1.0 mm of movement on blinking.

The lens size is determined from a table that relates the lens size to the base curve, ranging from 8.8 to 9.6 mm in size. Centration is somewhat dependent on size. Reducing the size of a lens with an apical bubble will improve centration, whereas increasing the size will reduce excessive movement and improve centration of a loose lens. If the larger lens is not sufficient to reduce the excessive movement and low riding, use of a minus carrier lenticular design will allow the upper lid to grasp the lens and raise it. Use of the steepest base curve and smallest lens size that would allow good centration and adequate movement are the goals to be achieved for the best lens fit.

Over-refraction is carried out monocularly for distant vision, using a phoropter or trial frame. For the near refraction, a trial frame should be used, adding +0.25-diopter lenses until the patient can read the finest print of the near-vision card. At this time the distant vision should still be good. Also, +0.50-diopter lenses should be added in order to blur the distant vision. If more plus power is necessary for near vision, a lens 0.05 mm steeper or a lens 0.1 mm steeper in a smaller size may be satisfactory.

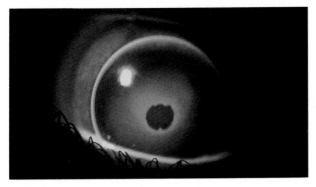

Fig. 6.33 *Tight aspheric rigid bifocal—apical bubble.*

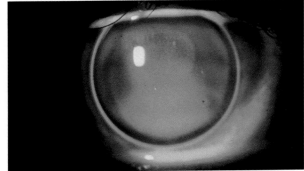

Fig. 6.34 *Tight aspheric rigid bifocal—peripheral touch.*

BIFOCAL AND MULTIFOCAL CONTACT LENSES

A lens is ordered, recognizing that it will often be necessary to order more than one pair of lenses. After receiving the lens, a period of 3–4 days or longer is necessary for the wearer to adapt to the lens as well as to "learn" to achieve the best vision.

Other gas-permeable or hard aspheric simultaneous-vision lenses are fit in a similar fashion. The individual fitting manual is required for the details of each lens.

PROBLEM SOLVING Power changes and poor centering or fit require the ordering of new lenses, utilizing the modification principles utilized in the fitting described above (Table 6.17). Before changing lenses it is good to allow sufficient time for the patient to become adapted to the lens, since the vision may improve during the first 1–2 weeks of wearing.

FRONT-SURFACE ASPHERIC SIMULTANEOUS-VISION LENSES
The fitting of these lenses is the same as that for any single-vision spherical lens (Fig. 6.35).

SOFT BIFOCAL LENSES
These lenses (Table 6.18) can be used only with less than 1.00 diopter of astigmatism and, depending on the specific lens, are available in limited parameters. The Barnes–Hind Hydrocurve II and the Bausch & Lomb P.A.I. bifocal lenses are examples of posterior aspheric bifocal lenses. The Hydrocurve II is much more effective in providing adequate bifocal power. Specific details must be obtained from each company.

TABLE 6.17 PROBLEM SOLVING
Too tight: Loosen
Too flat: Order new lens
Poor vision: Over-refract; order new lens; or convert to modified monovision or different lens type

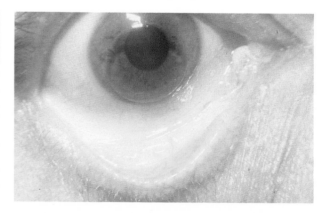

Fig. 6.35 *Front hard aspheric bifocal (Salvatori).*

BIFOCAL AND MULTIFOCAL CONTACT LENSES

The Hydrocurve II lens (Fig. 6.36) is available from +4.00 to -6.00 diopters, with an add up to +1.50 diopters, whereas the P.A.I. has sphere powers of +6.00 to -6.00 diopters.

The Ciba Bi-Soft lens (Fig. 6.37) is a soft lens with a central distance zone and a peripheral concentric near add, whereas the Alges bifocal has the reverse—a central near zone with a peripheral distance zone.

The above lenses are fit in a similar manner (see Table 6.17) (see Alges below for its fitting procedure): placing a lens, close to the subjective refraction, on the eye and allowing it to settle for 15–20 min. Adequate centration over the pupil is essential, with no more than 0.5–1.0-mm displacement of the lens on blinking. If movement is greater than this, the central distance zone may not consistently center over the pupil, thereby giving unacceptable visual acuity.

Over-refraction is carried out monocularly with hand-held lenses to get the distant-vision prescription. Caution must be exercised to make sure the near zone is not being over-refracted. After adding +0.50 diopter to blur the distant vision, -0.25-diopter lenses are added sparingly until vision is clear, using the

TABLE 6.18 SOFT BIFOCAL LENSES	
Diagnostic lens: Choose according to guidebook	Base curve: According to guidebook
Power: Spectacle refraction	Size: According to guidebook
	Over-refract

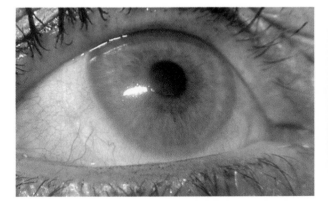

Fig. 6.36 *Hydrocurve II soft bifocal (Barnes–Hind).*

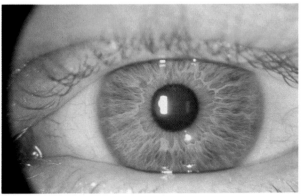

Fig. 6.37 *Bi-Soft bifocal (Ciba).*

BIFOCAL AND MULTIFOCAL CONTACT LENSES

minimum amount of minus possible. This lens power is then ordered.

Delivery of the lens is the same as other soft lenses, informing the patients that a time period usually is necessary to adapt to the new vision. Vision may vary and often requires a compromise between distant and near vision. In many patients it is not possible to satisfy prolonged near-vision requirements. Flare at night should also be discussed, since this is bothersome to some patients and may require time for adaptation.

PROBLEM SOLVING The most serious problem is that of poor vision, usually for reading (Table 6.19). If this cannot be solved, another lens type must be considered, unless this can be solved by ordering a lens of different power or different base curve if the cause of poor vision is due to a poorly centering lens. Flatter lenses require a steeper base curve, whereas looser lenses require a flatter base curve.

MODIFIED BIFOCAL OR MODIFIED MONOVISION

If binocular vision is not satisfactory, two compromises are possible. Using the bifocal lenses on both eyes, more plus on one eye than the other (modified bifocal) may allow a greater depth of field for intermediate tasks (Figs. 6.38 and 6.39). Otherwise, one may use a bifocal on one eye for near vision and a single-vision lens on the other eye for distant vision (modified monovision).

The fitting and problem solving are the same as those used for single-vision lenses (if monovision is utilized) and for simultaneous-vision lenses (if modified monovision is utilized).

TABLE 6.19
PROBLEM SOLVING

Poor centration: Change base curve accordingly
Poor vision: Over-refract; if not improved, choose alternative lens correction
Poor comfort: Choose alternative lens correction

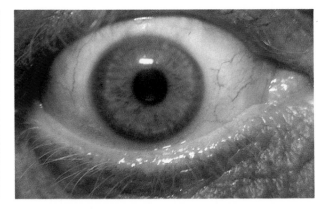

Fig. 6.38 *Modified monovision (right eye)—distant-vision single-vision soft tint (Ciba).*

ALGES SOFT LENS

This lens (Figs. 6.40 and 6.41; Table 6.20), with a central near portion and a peripheral distance portion, works on the simultaneous fitting principle and is fit from a fitting set. It is available in two base curves (8.60 and 8.90 mm), with distant powers of +6.00 to −6.00 diopters and add powers of +2.00 to +3.50 diopters. The add-segment diameters are 2.12, 2.35, or 2.55 mm.

The recommended starting point for fitting is: 8.90-mm base curve, 2.35-mm add segment, +2.50-diopter add power, and the appropriate distance power. The add-power requirement is somewhat dependent on the size of the add segment, with less power over the spectacle add being required with larger add segments. It should never be necessary to use more than 1.00

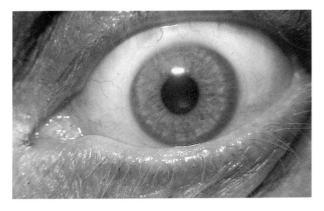

Fig. 6.39 *Modified monovision (left eye)—near-vision Bi-Soft bifocal (Ciba).*

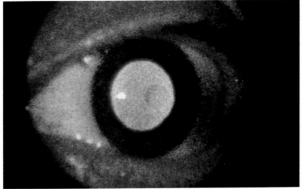

Fig. 6.40 *Alges soft bifocal (University Optical Products) shown in position on eye.*

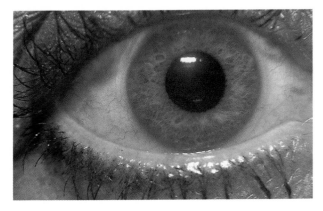

Fig. 6.41 *Alges soft bifocal lens.*

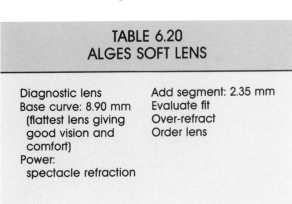

TABLE 6.20 ALGES SOFT LENS	
Diagnostic lens Base curve: 8.90 mm (flattest lens giving good vision and comfort) Power: spectacle refraction	Add segment: 2.35 mm Evaluate fit Over-refract Order lens

diopter over the spectacle add. With the 2.55-mm segment the required add in the contact lens will normally be the same as the spectacle add.

In general, perfect lens centration is not necessary for adequate function. Pupil size is not always relevant to add selection if some decentration of the segment occurs. Segment position and movement are evaluated best with an ophthalmoscope. Observe the red reflex, in which the segment is visible, by looking through the ophthalmoscope through about the +6.00- to +10.00-diopter lens (the black numbers) from a distance of about 6–10 inches. Avoid over-minusing for distance and tight lenses.

Aim for the flattest lens that provides good acuity and comfort with the largest add segment that does not interfere with distance vision in bright light. As with other lenses, explain the adaptation period so that the patient knows what to expect.

PROBLEM SOLVING Explanation of adaptation eliminates many problems (Table 6.21). Poor vision requires careful evaluation to determine a change of base curve or a change in the diameter of the near segment.

SYNSOFT SOFT BIFOCAL
This lens (Fig. 6.42) is an annular bifocal with a peripheral near portion surrounding the central distance zone; this lens works on the alternating-vision concept. Although no longer available, patients who have been wearing the lens successfully may present themselves to fitters.

A lens of the appropriate base curve and size is picked according to the table. It is then observed for adequate centration and movement. The lens should rest on the margin of the lower

TABLE 6.21 PROBLEM SOLVING
Poor vision: Modify base curve
Poor near vision: Vary segment size

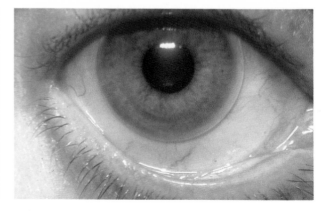

Fig. 6.42 *SynSoft soft bifocal (Salvatori).*

lid or just above this. With downgaze it should move upward about 2–3 mm. Over-refraction is carried out. The segment should be observed via the red reflex with the +6.00- to +10.00- diopter lens of the ophthalmoscope from about 6–10 inches away to be sure that the segment moves up adequately to a position slightly superior and temporal in the pupillary area. The distant portion should cover the superior two-thirds to three-quarters of the pupil.

If the lens is too tight or loose, it is changed appropriately. A flatter and/or smaller-diameter lens will fit more loosely, and a steeper and/or larger lens will be tighter.

PROBLEM SOLVING Poor vision is usually related to poor centering or movement, requiring (a) a looser lens to correct a high, tight lens or (b) a tighter lens to correct a low, loose lens. If not successful in improving vision, use an alternative lens type.

DURASOFT 2 SOFT BIFOCAL

This segmented lens (Fig. 6.43) is fit by choosing the appropriate lens from a four-lens diagnostic fitting set. The set has two pairs of lenses, one pair each of the high- and low-segment heights. There is one base curve (8.50 mm) and one diameter (13.5 mm). The lens must (a) be comfortable, (b) center well, and (c) translate adequately. An over-refraction is carried out for distant and near vision, often requiring a compromise between the two.

Over-refraction is carried out with a trial frame. Excessive movement requires a steeper lens, whereas a tight lens should be replaced by a looser one.

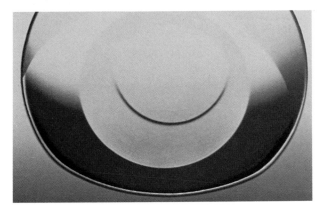

Fig. 6.43 *DuraSoft trufocal (Wesley Jessen).*

PROBLEM SOLVING If vision or comfort are not satisfactory, another type of vision correction should be chosen.

SOFTSITE OR BAUSCH & LOMB SEGMENTED BIFOCAL

These two lenses (Figs. 6.44 and 6.45) are fit in a similar manner, with the flatter-base-curve fitting lens being chosen for the 43.00–45.00-diopter corneas and the steeper-base-curve lens being chosen for the corneas steeper than 45.00 diopters. The spherical equivalent power lens +0.25 to +0.50 diopter is placed on the eye with the structural vent down. Distant over-refraction is performed. Because the patient has to undergo a learning phase, reading may not be easy at this time. If reading is not possible, go to a flatter lens. If still not possible, discontinue the fitting.

The lens must translate and move up 1–2 mm for reading. If poor gliding is encountered, use a flatter lens. With excessive movement, use a steeper lens. The lens must center adequately on the cornea, with the segment not going in front of the pupil during primary gaze or during blinking to avoid diplopia. The structural vent should be at 6 o'clock but may go up to 30° nasally or 10° temporally. The segment is seen more easily with the red reflex of the ophthalmoscope than with the slit lamp.

This lens may be used in conjunction with a single-vision lens in the modified monovision concept.

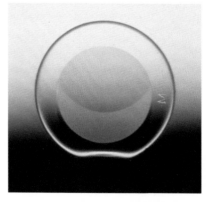 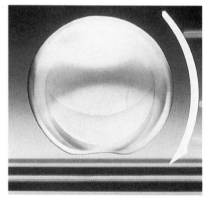

Fig. 6.44 *Softsite soft bifocal (Softsite contact lens laboratories).*

Fig. 6.45 *Crescent soft bifocal (Bausch & Lomb).*

PROBLEM SOLVING Poor vision and/or comfort requires choosing an alternative type of bifocal correction.

GENERAL PRINCIPLES FOR THE SOFT BIFOCALS

If adequate vision and centration cannot be obtained with the fitting set, it is best to refrain from ordering a lens. Although slight improvement may occur with time, it is not significant; much wasted time may be saved by not proceeding with these patients.

The realities of the best possible vision and limitations of the specific lens used should be discussed with the patient. These might be: glare, flare at night, second image with pupillary dilatation in dim illumination, compromised distant or near vision, discomfort of the lenses, lens care, limitations of the lens, etc. Discussion of these limitations beforehand will often allow patients to accept them and adjust well.

A patient may see extremely well with the diagnostic fitting lens but may not see as well when the final lens is ordered. Also, as time passes, especially with the soft lenses, the effectiveness of the add may decrease significantly. This may be because of a change in the optical characteristics of the lens or because of the need for increased add as a result of the patient being older.

As with any lenses, the risks of infection as well as tight signs and symptoms must be discussed, with the specifics of cleanliness and specific care regimens being stressed for all patients. The patient must be cautioned against choosing unknown solutions without checking with the fitter first. The fitter or someone responsible must be available at all times in case of problems, infection, etc. The patient must be instructed that if redness or pain of the eyes occurs, the lens should be removed immediately and the fitter or whoever is designated in case of an emergency should be contacted.

If bifocal soft lenses are not successful, it may be necessary to fit lenses by using the monovision technique; or perhaps the modified monovision technique should be considered if soft lenses are desired. If either of these are not successful, reading or bifocal spectacles may be worn over the single-vision distant contact lenses; or perhaps the fitter should consider fitting the patient with rigid bifocal lenses. If none of these are satisfactory, it may be necessary to discontinue contact lenses and wear spectacles.

RATE OF SUCCESS

The success (Figs. 6.46 and 6.47) rate varies considerably with the skill of the fitter and the lens type and design. The segmented hard and gas-permeable bifocals or monovision fitting can achieve a success rate of 70–80%. The aspheric simultaneous vision designs have a limited success rate and often function better as monovision lenses.

The segmented soft bifocals have had a poor success rate. The simultaneous soft bifocals have performed best as modified monovision lenses, except for the Alges and Hydrocurve II, which seem to have the most promise as a multifocal lens.

The parameters of success with regard to lens fitting are given in Table 6.22.

SUMMARY ON FITTING

If a patient has been wearing single-vision contact lenses for many years and develops the need for a presbyopic correction, it is often easiest to add a small amount of plus (or decrease minus) to one lens for reading or to fit the reading eye with a soft

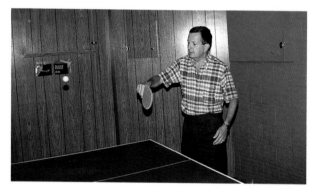

Fig. 6.46 *Photograph of the author wearing executive Boston IV bifocal while playing Ping-Pong.*

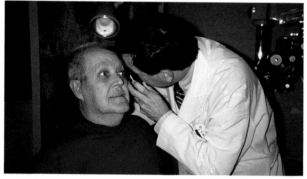

Fig. 6.47 *Photograph of the author wearing executive Boston IV bifocal while using an ophthalmoscope.*

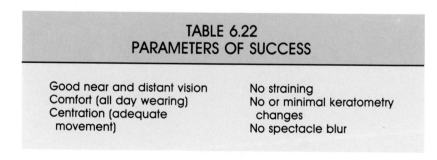

TABLE 6.22
PARAMETERS OF SUCCESS

Good near and distant vision	No straining
Comfort (all day wearing)	No or minimal keratometry
Centration (adequate	changes
movement)	No spectacle blur

simultaneous-vision lens (monovision or modified monovision).

If this is not tolerated or if the patient requires better binocular vision than has been obtained, a gas-permeable or hard bifocal lens may be used. If the patient has never worn contact lenses, start with a gas-permeable or hard bifocal. If a patient does not want a gas-permeable or hard lens, try one of the soft bifocals which has a better success rate or use the monovision or modified monovision method of fitting.

In summary, there are many types of bifocal lenses available (Table 6.23). The fitter must understand the difference between the alternating- and simultaneous-vision mechanisms and recognize the capabilities and limitations of each and explain these to the patient. Diagnostic fitting sets are recommended for all bifocal or multifocal contact lens fitting. Each specific lens will require a

TABLE 6.23
BIFOCAL CONTACT LENSES

DESIGN	TRADE NAME	MANUFACTURER	HARD	SOFT	RG-P	TYPE
NON-ASPHERICAL						
Nonsegmented	Bicon	Wesley-Jessen	XX			S
	Ve-Acc Translating	Vision-Ease			X	A
	Bivision	Vision-Ease			X	S
	Bisoft	CIBA		XX		S
	Alges	University Optical Products		XX	X	S
Segmented	Executive	Rooney Optical			XX	A
	Tangent-Streak	Fused Kontacts			XX	A
	One piece crescent segmented	Salvatori Ophthalmics			XX	A
	Fused cresent segmented	Many manufacturers	XX			A
	Softsite	Softsite		XX		A
	Cresent segment	Bausch & Lomb		XX		A
	Durasoft 2	Wesley-Jessen		XX		A
	Synsoft	Salvatori Ophthalmics		XX		A
ASPHERICAL						
Anterior	Vari-Range F	Precision Cosmet	XX			S
	Consta-Vue	Salvatori Ophthalmics	XX			S
Posterior	APA	GBF			XX	S
	VFL II	Conforma	XX			S
	Presbiflex	Breger/Mueller-Welt	XX			S
	Total-Vue	Quality Optics	XX			S
	PA I	Bausch & Lomb		XX		S
	Hydrocurve II	Barnes Hind		XX		S

separate fitting set and will have a fitting manual giving the available parameters and details of fitting. Many multifocal lenses work well, providing significant happiness for patients who require bifocal correction and wish to dispense with spectacles.

BIBLIOGRAPHY

1. Andrasko, G. J. Bifocal soft lenses: A comparison. *Contact Lens Forum,* 9:53–65, 1984.

2. Bailey, N. J. Contact lens update 1985. *Contract Lens Forum,* 9:43–44, 1985.

3. Boerner, C. F., and Thrasher, B. H. Results of monovision correction in bilateral pseudophakes. *Am. Intraocul. Implant. Soc. J.,* 10:49–51, 1984.

4. Capland, L., and Molinari, J. Clinical investigation of the Salvatori Sof-Form bifocal soft lens. *Int. Contact Lens Clin.,* 11:157–166, 1984.

5. Charman, W. N. Optical characteristics of Bausch and Lomb soflens (PAI) bifocals. *Int. Contact Lens Clin.,* 11:564–574, 1984.

6. Forst, G. Investigations into the stabilization of bifocal contact lenses. *Int. Contact Lens Clin.,* 14:68–75, 1987.

7. Goldberg, J. Aspheric multifocals' usable vision zone. *Contact Lens Forum,* 7:53–57, 1982.

8. Greco, A. *Int. Contact Lens Clin.,* 12:86–92, 1985.

9. Greco, A. New soft bifocals. *Int. Eyecare,* 2:128–132, 1986.

10. Hanks, A. Contact lenses for presbyopia. *Eye Contact,* 1:9–14, 1984.

11. Kreshon, M. Fitting the B & L bifocal soft lens. *Contact Lens Forum,* 8:49–56, 1983.

12. Magnuson, R. H. Variable focus hard contact lens. *Ophthalmology Times,* 2:3, 1977.

13. Maltzman, B., Harris, M., and Esby, J. Experience with soft bifocal lenses. *CLAO J.,* 11:73–77, 1985.

14. Weinstock, F. J. Aphakic patients can be happy with bifocal contact lenses. *Contact Lens Med. Bull.,* 7:63–65, 1974.

15. Weinstock, F. J., and Michaille, K. Aspheric multifocal contact lenses. *Contact Intraocul. Lens J.,* 5:90–92, 1979.

16. Weinstock, F. J. Alternatives available to the presbyope and aphake. *Contact Intraocul. Lens J.,* 5:93–95, 1979.

17. Weinstock, F. J. (Moderator). Symposium—Correction of presbyopia with contact lenses. *CLAO J.,* 11:255–273, 1985.

18. Weinstock, F. J. Correction of presbyopia. In: Dabezies, O. H., Jr. (Ed.). *Contact Lenses: The CLAO Guide to Basic Sciences and Clinical Practice,* pp. 57.1–57.18, Grune & Stratton, Orlando, Florida, 1986.

7

KERATOCONUS, CORNEAL TRANSPLANTS, AND IRREGULAR ASTIGMATISM

JOSEPH SOPER, F.C.L.S.A.

Fitting irregular corneal surfaces presents a significant challenge to the fitter. Because of surface irregularity, obtaining an adequate lens–cornea relationship is difficult. Rigid lenses frequently do not develop good capillary attraction and may displace partially or completely off the cornea and/or out of the eye. Large-diameter soft lenses may yield a satisfactory fit, but because of their tendency to mold to the more rigid underlying irregular surface, they usually do not provide acceptable optical correction for these eyes. This chapter will discuss the several types of irregular surfaces separately, since the approach to fitting each one is somewhat different.

KERATOCONUS

The classic textbook line drawing of keratoconus shown in Fig. 7.1 illustrates the change from a normal corneal thickness and topography (in the shaded area) to that of the conelike central corneal protrusion and the thinning of the keratoconus cornea. The challenge in fitting such a surface with a rigid corneal lens is to fit the steep central area and the surrounding flatter zone simultaneously with the same lens.

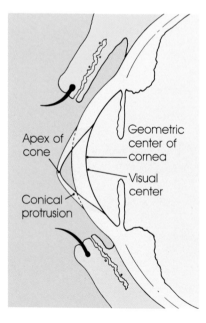

Fig. 7.1 *Contact lens must bridge over the conical protrusion.*

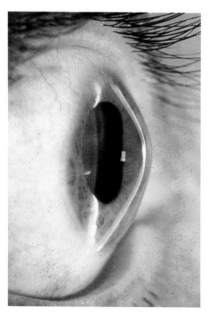

Fig. 7.2 *Profile view of keratonconus.*

Fig. 7.3 *Ideal contact-lens–cornea relationship in keratoconus.*

The profile view of a keratoconus cornea in Fig. 7.2 illustrates the scarring in the apex of the cornea which produces additional irregularity in the surface. The epithelium over the central apex, especially when thinning and scarring have developed, often is compromised and will show varying degrees of superficial punctate keratitis (S.P.K.). In fitting the contact lens, it is imperative to bridge over this area to ensure that no trauma is created by the lens (1). Theories stating that pressure on the apex by the lens forestalls conical development are not well founded. Conversely, apical pressure will more likely cause increased scarring and thinning (2).

The ideal lens–cornea relationship is shown in Fig. 7.3. This illustration shows a rigid lens that bridges the apex of the cone while being significantly flatter in the peripheral zone. The bearing point of lens touch in such a lens is in the intermediate zone, between the center and the edge of the lens. This type of lens fitting produces a lens that centers directly over the apex of the cone. If the cone is displaced away from the geometric center of the cornea, which is the most frequent positioning, the lens will displace in the same location. Frequently the well-fitted lens in this condition will be found to locate itself grossly away from the geometric center of the cornea. Attempts to refit such a case to produce "better centering" will lead to a totally unacceptable lens–cornea relationship.

The keratoconus lens, when viewed as in Fig. 7.4, shows a steep central zone that fits over the conical apex and is surrounded by a flatter area. Both of these areas are lathe cut and polished separately on the back surface of a lens blank in the manufacturing process. This is not a modification to a previously finished lens.

A diagnostic set of keratoconus lenses (shown in Fig. 7.5) consists of lenses that have increasing vaulting effect from front

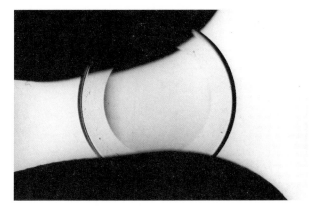

Fig. 7.4 *Keratonconus contact lens.*

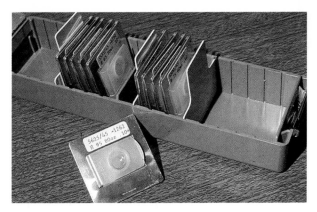

Fig. 7.5 *Diagnostic contact lens fitting set.*

MANAGEMENT OF CORNEAL IRREGULARITIES WITH CONTACT LENSES

to back of the set (3). Diagnostic lenses are used to determine the fitting parameters of the lens to be specified for the patient.

The change in the vaulting effect by varying the diameter of the steep center zone is illustrated in Fig. 7.6. The lenses depicted all have the same central and peripheral zone *curvatures* but have increasingly larger central zone *diameters*. The lens on the right will demonstrate significantly more vaulting than that on the left. Changing the central zone diameter of a lens by 1.0 mm, while maintaining the same central posterior curvature and lens diameter, increases the vaulting effect of the lens equal to steepening the curvature by 10 diopters, whereas small changes (1 diopter) in curvature will create only minor fitting changes.

Vaulting effect can be better described as the "sagittal value" of a lens. This is depicted in Fig. 7.6 as the distance between the posterior apex of the lens and the vertical straight line between the edges of the CPC diameter. The diagnostic set of lenses in Fig. 7.5 were designed to produce a controlled gradual increase in sagittal value, as shown in Table 7.1. All the specifications of each lens are shown, and most importantly the sagittal-value changes from one lens to the next are enumerated. The fitter, when departing from the listed lenses and wishing to change a lens parameter (CPC diameter or radius), should know what change in sagittal value will be created.

Keratometry is of little value in determining the final specifications of a patient's lens, since the keratometer only measures truly spherical surfaces (such as ball bearings) and cannot measure a conical surface as on a keratoconus cornea (4). When

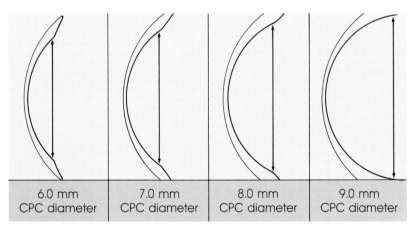

| 6.0 mm CPC diameter | 7.0 mm CPC diameter | 8.0 mm CPC diameter | 9.0 mm CPC diameter |

Fig. 7.6 *Vaulting effect ("sagittal value" of lens) in relation to diameter of the steep center zone.*

measuring a cone the instrument will indicate a "reading" which is interpreted as if it were a sphere. The reading obtained is only valuable in comparing one cone to another and in categorizing each cone as early, advanced, or severe. These classifications are related to the keratometer readings given in Table 7.2. The main value of the K-reading in fitting the patient is to aid in the choice of the *first* diagnostic lens to be tried. If the measurement indicates an early cone, the first lens tried would be one with a small sagittal value; however, if the readings indicate a severe cone, the first lens would be one with a large sagittal value (5).

The first lens tried is evaluated with fluorescein and a slit lamp. The relationship between the lens vaulting effect and the

TABLE 7.1
SOPER KERATOCONUS DIAGNOSTIC LENS SET

Sagittal Depth (mm)	CPC (diopters)	Power (diopters)	Lens Diameter (mm)	Thickness (mm)	Diameter of CPC (mm)
0.68	48/45	− 4.50	7.5	0.10	6.0
0.73	52/45	− 8.50	7.5	0.10	6.0
0.80	56/45	− 12.50	7.5	0.10	6.0
0.87	60/45	− 16.50	7.5	0.10	6.0
1.00	52/45	− 8.50	8.5	0.10	7.0
1.12	56/45	− 12.50	8.5	0.10	7.0
1.22	60/45	− 16.50	8.5	0.10	7.0
1.37	52/45	− 8.50	9.5	0.10	8.0
1.52	56/45	− 12.50	9.5	0.10	8.0
1.67	60/45	− 16.50	9.5	0.10	8.0

TABLE 7.2
CLASSIFICATION OF THE DEGREE OF CONICAL PROGRESSION BY USE OF K-READING

EARLY CONE:	SEVERE CONE:	ADVANCE CONE:
48.00–52.00	56.00 and higher	52.00–56.00

cone is observed. If the vaulting is excessive, a bubble will be trapped between the lens and the cornea as shown in Fig. 7.7. This will indicate that a lens with less sagittal value should be tried.

A lens with inadequate vaulting is shown in Fig. 7.8. It demonstrates a gross apical touch, since no fluorescein-stained tear is found between the CPC and apex of the cone. A diagnostic lens with greater sagittal value should be tried.

The diagnostic lens that shows apical clearance with circulation of fluorescein-stained tear beneath it without entrapping air is the "best-fit" lens, as shown in Fig. 7.9. A *spherical* refraction is performed over the best diagnostic lens to determine the power needed for the patient's lens. The power of the over-refraction is added directly to that of the diagnostic lens. Cylinders *are not* included in the over-refraction, since the patient's

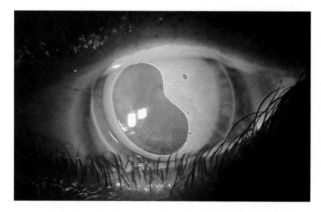

Fig. 7.7 *Excessive vaulting with trapped bubble.*

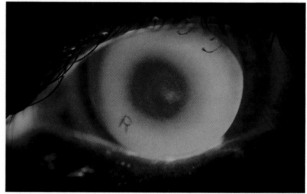

Fig. 7.8 *Inadequate vaulting with apical touch.*

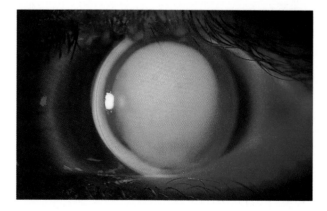

Fig. 7.9 *"Best-fit" lens with apical clearance and good fluorescein circulation.*

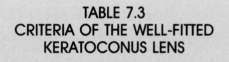

TABLE 7.3
CRITERIA OF THE WELL-FITTED KERATOCONUS LENS

1. Apical clearance without lens-induced S.P.K.
2. Maximum obtainable visual acuity
3. All-waking-hours wearing time

lens can only be made in a spherical configuration. Adding cylinder to the patient's lens would require prism and/or other stabilization methods which would adversely affect the lens "fit." After the patient's lens is received and it is found that a significant cylinder is required to obtain best visual acuity, spectacles should be prescribed with cylinder to be worn in conjunction with the contact lens.

The criteria of the well-fitted lens for keratoconus are shown in Table 7.3.

KERATOPLASTY

The cornea that has received a corneal graft presents several areas of significantly different topographies: the central donor graft, the peripheral host, and the raised scarred graft–host junction. If a smooth apposition of the graft and the host exists for a complete 360°, fitting contact lenses may not be complicated. When the graft–host junction has different elevations, as shown in Fig. 7.10, the fitting of a contact lens can become very difficult (6). In such cases the lens tends to displace toward the graft–host junction. To overcome lens decentration, large lenses are required.

Lens diameters ranging in size from 9.0 to 11.0 mm may be required to fit grafted corneas. A diagnostic set of larger-diameter lenses (Fig. 7.11) is used to determine the "best fit." These lenses need to be in phakic as well as aphakic powers. The diagnostic set needs to be rather larger in number, because both very flat and steep lenses are required. Keratometer readings are of min-

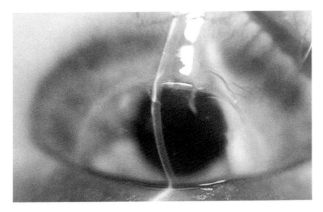

Fig. 7.10 *Graft–host junction with different elevations.*

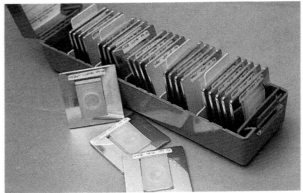

Fig. 7.11 *Keratoplasty diagnostic fitting lens set (larger-diameter lenses).*

MANAGEMENT OF CORNEAL IRREGULARITIES WITH CONTACT LENSES

imal value because they only relate to a small central area of the graft and ignore the balance of the corneal surface. K-readings are only valuable as a "starting place" and may not have any bearing on the final specifications of the patient's lens.

The diameter of the first lens selected is a mean of those available in the set while the CPC is near K. After the diagnostic lens is inserted, fluorescein is added to the eye, and the lens–cornea relationship is evaluated with the aid of a slit lamp. The lens may displace in one direction and override the limbus (Fig. 7.12); if so, a lens of steeper CPC and/or larger diameter is the next diagnostic lens tried. If the lens has large stationary bubbles trapped over the graft, a lens with less vaulting effect (i.e., smaller and/or flatter) would be tried. A number of diagnostic lenses may need to be tried before finding the most suitable fit. A *spherical* refraction is done over the best-fitting diagnostic lens to determine the power of the lens to be ordered for the patient.

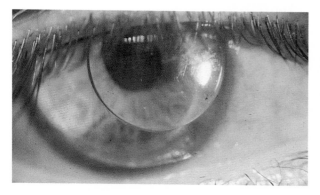

Fig. 7.12 *Displacement with overriding of limbus (flat lens).*

Fig. 7.13 *Optimal fit—post-keratoplasty.*

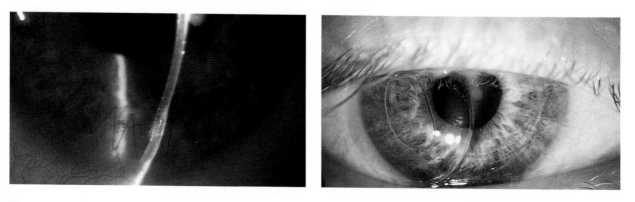

Fig. 7.14 *Flat graft (poor candidate for rigid lens).*

Fig. 7.15 *"Best-fit" rigid lens on a flat graft.*

MANAGEMENT OF CORNEAL IRREGULARITIES WITH CONTACT LENSES

An optimal fit (Fig. 7.13) is demonstrated by a lens that is exhibiting a bearing on the host portion of the cornea and resting gently on the graft–host junction while vaulting over the graft.

Rigid lenses, under certain circumstances, will not function regardless of the number of diagnostic lenses tried. Typical in this regard are lenses applied to *flat grafts* in which the graft is sunken as compared to the surrounding host, as shown in Fig. 7.14.

When a flat graft is present, the steepest point on the corneal surface becomes the graft–host junction. As a rule, all rigid lenses tend to center over the steeper point on the cornea. Figure 7.15 shows the "best-fit" rigid lens on a flat graft. This lens, though, is unacceptable because it displaces half onto the sclera, exposes half of the pupil, and traps a large bubble under its geometric center. In such a case, better lens centering could only be accomplished by a larger lens diameter and/or a steeper CPC. Either change would increase the lens vaulting effect and thereby increase the size of the trapped air bubble.

In cases of fitting corneal grafts where rigid lenses totally decenter, fitting piggy back (soft and hard) lenses has proved very successful (7). This lens system is demonstrated in Fig. 7.16, which shows a flat graft over which is fitted a large-diameter *aphakic* soft lens and a steep rigid lens. The rigid lens is necessary to optically neutralize the irregular astigmatism on the anterior surface of the soft lens. The soft lens needs to be an aphakic lens to provide a steep surface over which the rigid lens can be fitted; otherwise, the rigid lens would displace as it did over the corneal surface. Aphakic soft lenses are used even if the eye being fitted is phakic.

The eye in Fig. 7.15 is shown refitted with a piggy-back system in Fig. 7.17. The rigid lens centers directly over the apex of the front surface of the aphakic soft lens.

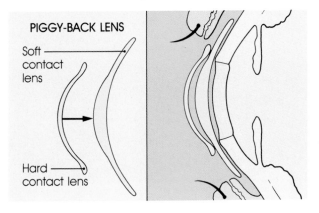

Fig. 7.16 *Piggy-back lens concept.*

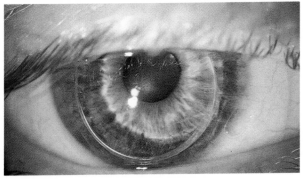

Fig. 7.17 *Piggy-back lens on flat cornea (refit of Fig. 7.15).*

The power of the lenses to be supplied to the patient is determined by a *spherical* over-refraction of the diagnostic piggy-back lenses. The power of the patient's aphakic soft lens should be the same as the diagnostic lens, whereas the power of the patient's rigid lens will be calculated by adding the spherical over-refraction directly to that of the rigid diagnostic lens. Patient care and handling of the piggy-back lenses are the same as that for each of the two types of systems being used. The piggy-back system can also be used in fitting keratoconus patients who cannot tolerate a rigid lens (8) (Fig. 7.18).

Fig. 7.18 *Piggy-back lens on keratoconus patient who could not tolerate a rigid lens.*

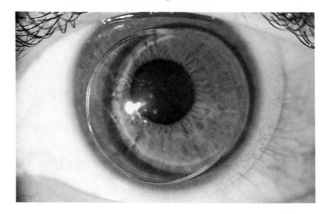

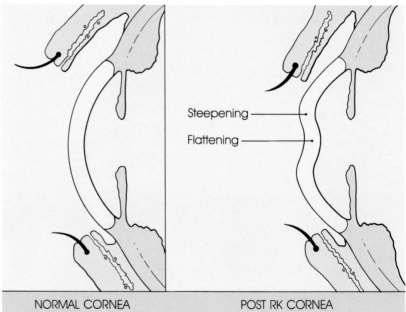

Fig. 7.19 *Comparison of normal cornea with post-R.K. cornea.*

RADIAL KERATOTOMY

The intended topographical changes to the cornea following radial keratotomy (R.K.) are a flattening of the central apex of the cornea while steepening the peripheral zone (Fig. 7.19). This configuration presents a contact lens fitting problem not unlike that of the flat graft, with the tendency of the lens to displace over the steep peripheral zone (Fig. 7.20).

Keratometry also presents the same problems as in keratoplasty and therefore is of little value as an aid in contact lens fitting. The best fitting approach is to use the preoperative K-readings as a starting place for trying diagnostic lenses (9). The same diagnostic set used for fitting keratoplasty is utilized; the final lens most frequently will be large in diameter to obtain best centering. If the lens rides high under the top lid (Fig. 7.21),

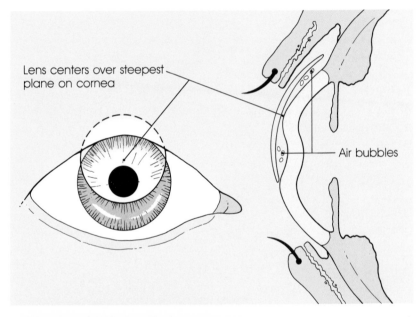

Lens centers over steepest plane on cornea

Air bubbles

Fig. 7.20 *High-riding contact lens on post-R.K. cornea.*

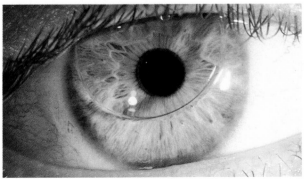

Fig. 7.21 *High-riding contact lens on post-R.K. cornea. This situation requires prism ballasting.*

prism ballasting may be necessary in order to add weight to the bottom of the lens so the lens will move downward.

A spherical refraction is done over the best-fitting diagnostic lens to determine the power of the patient's lens.

Soft lenses are contraindicated for R.K. according to Ira Shivitz, M.D. (9). He reported neovascularization of 14 corneas from 23 eyes fitted with soft lenses following R.K., while none fitted with rigid lenses developed neovascularization.

TRAUMATIC IRREGULAR ASTIGMATISM

Corneas with irregular astigmatism secondary to trauma as shown in Fig. 7.22 present the same lens-fitting problems as those discussed for keratoconus and keratoplasty. The fitting techniques are exactly the same, entailing diagnostic lens evaluation. K-readings are of little value but can be used as a starting place for the diagnostic lens fitting system. A rigid lens may be found that will fit adequately; however, if such a lens cannot be found, a piggy-back fitting is indicated. A soft lens by itself is contraindicated because of its inadequate optical correction of the irregular astigmatism.

LENS MATERIALS

In all fittings discussed herein, the patient's rigid lenses are fabricated from the most highly oxygen-permeable material available. Consideration is also given to the performance qual-

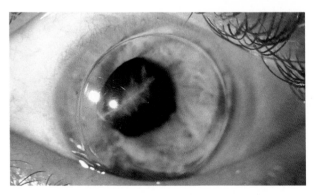

Fig. 7.22 *Irregular astigmatism secondary to trauma.*

TABLE 7.4 REQUIRED PROPERTIES OF LENS MATERIAL
1. Lens materials for both rigid and soft lenses must be highly oxygen permeable
2. Soft lenses must withstand deterioration due to daily handling

ities of the material to be prescribed (i.e., optics, stability, and surface integrity). The soft lens for the piggy-back lenses likewise should be of high oxygen permeability but must not be so fragile as to be damaged as a result of daily handling (Table 7.4).

THE SATURN LENS

The Saturn lens holds promise for the fitting of keratoconus, keratoplasty, radial keratotomy, and traumatic irregular astigmatism (8). This lens, shown in Fig. 7.23, is manufactured using both soft (HEMA) and rigid (Styrene) materials. The peripheral portion is soft, and the central zone is of oxygen-permeable rigid material. The advantage of this lens for the conditions discussed herein is its ability to present good lens centering and comfort, because of its soft lens characteristics. It also has the ability to supply a quality of optical correction equal to that of rigid lenses as well as provide gas transmissibility of gas-permeable rigid lenses.

Figure 7.24 shows a corneal graft that has been fitted with a Saturn lens, whereas Fig. 7.25 shows a keratoconus patient with

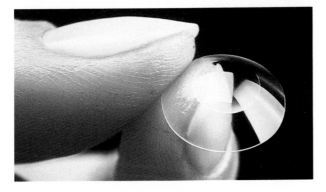

Fig. 7.23 *Saturn lens.*

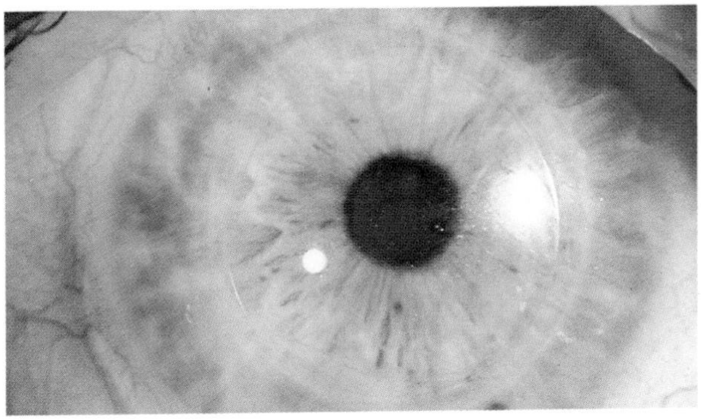

Fig. 7.24 *Corneal graft fit with Saturn lens.*

Fig. 7.25 *Keratoconus patient fit with Saturn lens.*

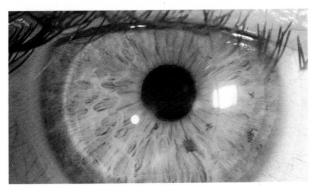

this lens. A patient with radial keratotomy, otherwise unable to be fitted with rigid lenses, is shown wearing a Saturn lens in Fig. 7.26. Eyes with a traumatic irregular astigmatism can also be fitted with a Saturn lens.

The fitting procedure is to take a K-reading to be used as a starting place. A diagnostic lens from a diagnostic set of lenses (Fig. 7.27) is chosen to match the flattest K-reading. Large-molecular fluorescein is instilled, and using a slit lamp the lens–cornea relationship is evaluated. Bubbles beneath the center of the lens indicate too great a vault, and the next-flattest lens is tried. If apical touch is observed, the lens–cornea relationship indicates insufficient vaulting. The next-steepest lens from the diagnostic set is then tried. In most cases all diagnostic lenses will show good centering due to their large diameter, which allows for the soft portion of the lens to fit beyond limbus onto the sclera. Patient comfort and good visual acuity have been obtained with the Saturn lens in these difficult cases.

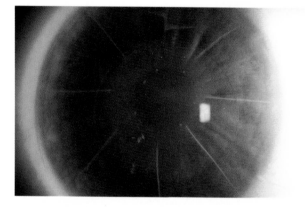

Fig. 7.26 *Radial keratotomy patient (unable to wear rigid lens) fit with Saturn lens.*

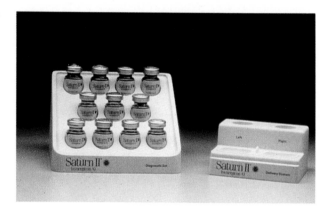

Fig. 7.27 *Saturn lens diagnostic fitting set.*

REFERENCES

1. Ridley, F. *Corneal and Scleral Lenses*, p. 112. Mosby, St. Louis, 1967.

2. Girard, L. J., Soper, J. W., and Sampson, W. G. *Corneal Contact Lenses*, 1st edition, p. 306. Mosby, St. Louis, 1967.

3. Soper, J. W., and Jarrett, A. Results of a systematic approach to fitting keratoconus and corneal transplants. *Contact Lens J.*, 2:3, 1975.

4. Soper, J. W. *Contact Lens Forum*, 2:25–32, 1977.

5. Buxton, J. N. *Corneal and Scleral Contact Lenses*, p. 116. Mosby, St. Louis, 1967.

6. Soper, J. W. Fitting corneal transplants with corneal contact lenses. *Int. Contact Lens Clin.*, 3(1):31–35, 1976.

7. Soper, J. W., and Paton, D. A piggy back contact lens system for corneal transplants and other cases with high astigmatism. *Contact Intraocul. Lens Med. J.* 6(2):132–143, 1980.

8. Soper, J. W. Fitting keratoconus with piggy back and saturn II lenses. *Contact Lens Forum*, 11:25–30, 1986.

9. Shivitz, I. A. Optical correction of postoperative radial keratotomy patients with contact lenses. *CLAO J.* 12(1):59–62, 1986.

8
TINTED SOFT LENSES: THE FULL SPECTRUM

LEROY G. MESHEL, M.D.

Soon after Dr. Otto Wichterle realized the potential of polyhydroxyethyl methacrylate (PHEMA) for forming gel contact lenses, he described several methods for imparting color additives to these lenses (1,2). Commercial tinting of soft contact lenses, however, is a relatively new phenomenon in contact lens manufacturing (3–5).

Unlike hard contact lenses, the original interest in tinting soft contact lenses was for prosthetics (6,7).

INDICATIONS

Soft contact lenses are now tinted for one (or more) of the following six reasons:

1. Visualization: Minimal overall lens tinting aids in seeing the lenses in a holding centration.
2. Informational: Imprinting data on the lens provides information beneficial to lens dispensers and wearers.
3. Fashion tinting: Contact lenses can enhance, modify, or change eye color.
4. Prosthetics: Prosthetic soft lenses are used to improve the cosmetic appearance and/or the visual function of an abnormal eye.
5. Experimentation: Tinted lenses have been used in many biologic experimental programs.
6. Specialty lenses: Tinted lenses designed for an unusual specific function.

Tinting for all these purposes will be discussed in this chapter.

Fig. 8.1 *Opaque and translucent lenses on mock dark eye. Note effects of the different types of lenses.*

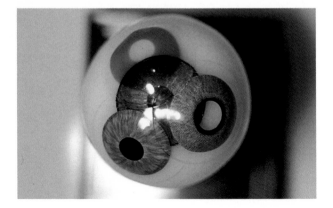

TINTED SOFT LENSES: THE FULL SPECTRUM

LENS TYPES

Generally speaking, tinted lenses are either translucent or opaque (Fig. 8.1).

TRANSLUCENT TINTED LENS

A translucent lens is transparent. Tinting modifies the color characteristics of light passing through the lens, but light is refractively undisturbed. The apparent iris color results from the tint of the contact lens and the color of the underlying iris or cornea (Fig. 8.2). The pupillary area of the lens can be the same color (e.g., sunshade lenses), clear, or have a black center for prosthetic pupillary imagery. This type of lens is particularly useful in enhancing or modifying eye color and in covering corneal leukomas. Translucent lenses are ineffective in disguising a dark-colored abnormality of the anterior eye or in changing eye color from a darker shade to a lighter shade (e.g., brown to blue).

OPAQUE TINTED LENS

In an opaque lens, the iris imagery is placed on an opaque substrate. Such lenses essentially project only their own imagery. The underlying cornea and iris are not seen. The resultant eye

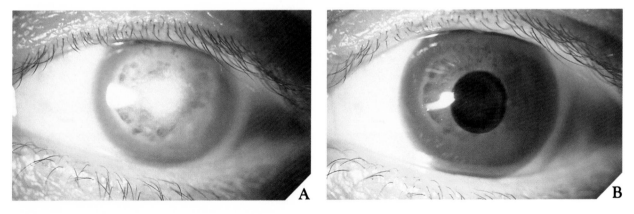

Fig. 8.2 (A) *Postcorneal tattoing with pigment migration.* (B) *Translucent cosmetic lens over corneal scar results in excellent imagery.*

OPAQUE TINTING

To produce an opaque lens, four methods are currently being used. Titmus Euracon was the first manufacturer to develop opaque soft contact lenses. Using a gravure process and opaque inks, they printed an iris image on a dome of clear PHEMA. They repolymerized clear PHEMA on top of the dome and lathe cut a "sandwich" opaque lens (Fig. 8.5). The lens was then hydrated. Wesley–Jessen Corporation utilized the same process but printed a dot matrix pattern on the anterior surface of the lens. (9) (Fig. 8.6). They were the first to gain U.S.F.D.A. approval for an opaque soft contact lens. Charles Neefe developed a method of doping PHEMA with titanium dioxide or ground oyster shells (calcium carbonate). A ring of this opaque PHEMA is used as a core around which is repolymerized clear PHEMA. The dry lens is cut from this button. At the Narcissus Foundation, Meshel and Presley have devised laser methods for opacification of the PHEMA matrix. Meshel and Gregory have devised a chemical precipitation method for lens opacification.

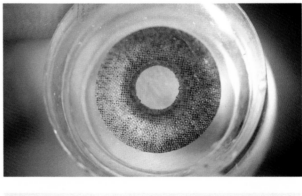

Fig. 8.5 *Titmus Euracon lens button before lathing the lens.*

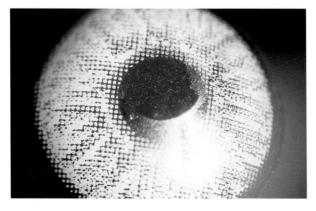

Fig. 8.6 *Wesley–Jessen opaque cosmetic lens.*

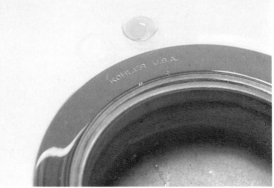

Fig. 8.7 *Visualization tint. (Courtesy of Ciba CLC.)*

INDICATIONS FOR TINTING SOFT CONTACT LENSES

VISUALIZATION TINTING

As with rigid lenses, a light overall tint enables the wearer to find the lens in a storage or cleaning container. This feature has become popular with the consumer and therefore has become a selling point for the marketers of soft contact lenses. Tints are usually light blue or green (Fig. 8.7).

Acid-reactive dyes have proven susceptible to fading, especially after exposure to chlorinated compounds during recreation or cleaning.

INFORMATIONAL TINTING

Tinting is useful for placing identifying information on a soft lens [e.g., manufacturer's logo, lens parameters (base curve, power)] or for marking the base of a prism-ballasted toric lens. This has been helpful for diagnostic fitting of lenses and for patient convenience (Fig. 8.8).

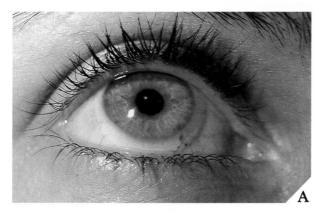 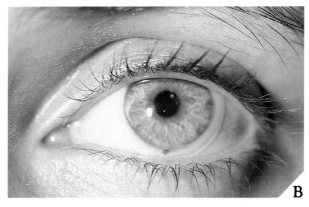

Fig. 8.8 *Diagnostic toric lens fitting utilizing tinted mark at base of prism. (A) Mark is ro-* *tated 45° nasally. (B) Prism-ballasted lens is centering well with mark at 6 o'clock.*

The author and Mr. Vernon Gregory invented a device, now produced by Barnes–Hind Corporation, which allows the lens dispenser to imprint a tiny "R" or "L" on any soft lens. This allows the lens wearer to distinguish between the right and and left lenses and to determine if either of these lenses is inverted (Fig. 8.9).

FASHION TINTING

Almost all of the major manufacturers now produce fashion-tinted translucent lenses for the modification of eye color (Fig. 8.10). International Hydron Corporation provides a device that

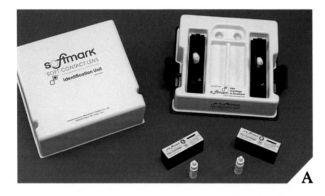
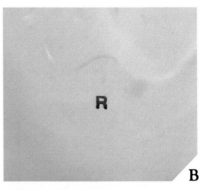

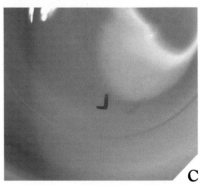

Fig. 8.9 (A) *Softmark "R" and "L" imprinter. (B) The "R" is in the correct orientation; therefore the lens is correctly oriented. (C) The "L" is reversed; therefore the lens is inverted.*

Fig. 8.10 *Fashion tint lens for modification of eye color—translucent type.*

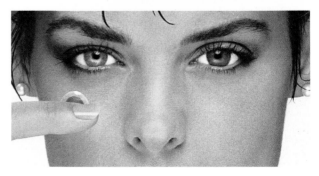

allows individual labs or dispensers to impart translucent fashion tints to soft lenses.

PROSTHETIC CONTACT LENSES

With the introduction of clear soft contact lenses in the United States in the early 1960s, it became apparent that this type of lens would be an ideal carrier for prosthetic imagery. The lenses covered the entire cornea and a portion of the sclera. They were comfortable and could be worn for long periods of time. Because of these fitting characteristics, prosthetic soft lenses tracked well with the globe and imparted a more realistic appearance, as compared to large immobile scleral stents in non- or semi-physical eyes (Fig. 8.11).

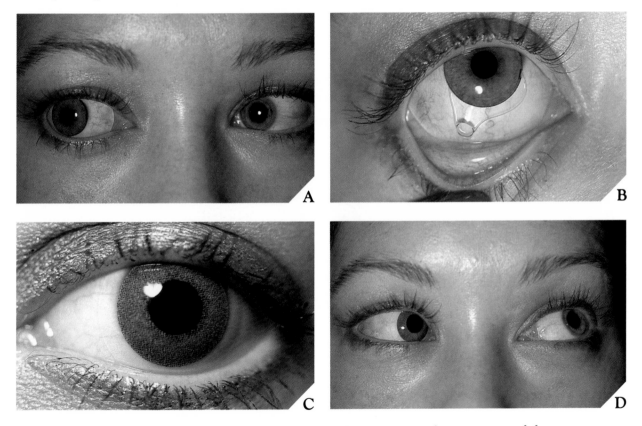

Fig. 8.11 *Corneal stent versus cosmetic soft lens. Note how realistically the soft prosthetic lens tracks. (A) Corneal stent on nonphthisic right eye. Note poor tracking and apparent buphthalmos on* right. (B) *Corneal stent one nonphthisic eye; poor comfort. (C) Soft prosthetic contact lens on same eye as (B); comfortable with good tracking. (D) Soft prosthetic lens; comfortable with good tracking.*

DESIGN

In general, the least amount of tint imagery necessary to produce maximum cosmetic effect is utilized (Fig. 8.12). The type of lens provided depends on the problem presented. (See indications for prosthetic lenses.) Initially, for precautionary purposes, the greatest percentage of patients fit with tinted prosthetic lenses had disfigured nonseeing eyes (e.g., corneal leukomas). Translucent imagery was the preferred method for prosthetic fabrication. Recent experience has demonstrated a shift toward the production and dispensing of opaque prosthetic lenses for both seeing and blind eyes.

Translucent prosthetic lenses are currently available in any refractive power, including high degrees of astigmatic correction. Opaque lenses are available in a full range of spherical refractive

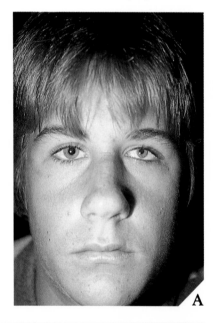

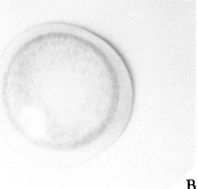

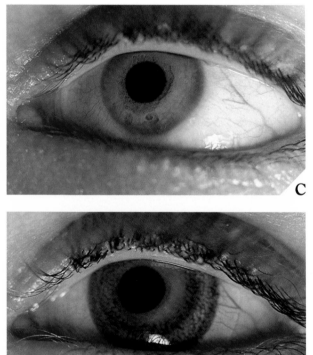

Fig. 8.12 *Minimal lens tinting to camouflage a microphthalmic eye. (A) Patient with microphthalmic left eye. (B) Minimally tinted soft prosthetic lens. (C) Microphthalmic eye without lens. (D) Microphthalmic eye with soft prosthetic lens.*

power and are available with astigmatic correction.

For correction of astigmatic refractive errors and for optimal cosmetic improvement of deviated eyes (exo-, eso-, or hyper-deviated), prism-ballasted lenses are used as a substrate for prosthetic imagery. Prism-ballasted soft contact lenses can effectively carry displaced prosthetic imagery. This type of prosthesis can compensate for distortion or displacement of the cornea or globe. Displaced imagery therefore makes a strabismic eye look more orthophoric. Any soft lens can be used as a carrier of prosthetic imagery (Fig. 8.13). High-water-content lenses (e.g., 55–65% H_2O) is preferred, especially on disease-compromised eyes. Studies performed by Dr. Irving Fat at the University of California, Berkeley, have demonstrated no significant decrease in oxygen transport across these lenses after tinting. (10).

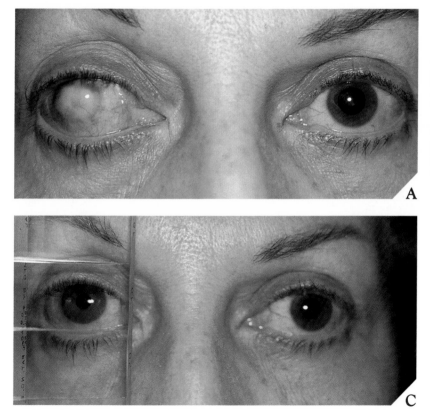

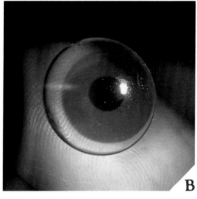

Fig. 8.13 Traumatic leukoma—exodeviation. Patient is made to look orthophoric by displacement of iris imagery on ballasted lens and by incorporating a prism in her spectacles. (A) Traumatized right eye with leukoma. (B) Prism ballast cosmetic lens with displaced imagery. (C) Patient wearing prosthetic lens with deviation corrected by prism.

INDICATIONS FOR TINTED PROSTHETIC SOFT CONTACT LENSES

Information for this section was derived from data obtained from the files of Narcissus Medical Research Foundation, Daly City, California (11). The indications for these lenses are categorized according to whether the eye is nonseeing or seeing. In an earlier series, 73% of lenses were dispensed for blind eyes (12); this percentage has lowered to about 50% of eyes fitted.

Fig. 8.14 *Buphthalmos.*

Fig. 8.15 (A) *Traumatic leukoma in patient without contact lens.* (B) *Patient wearing translucent prosthetic lens.*

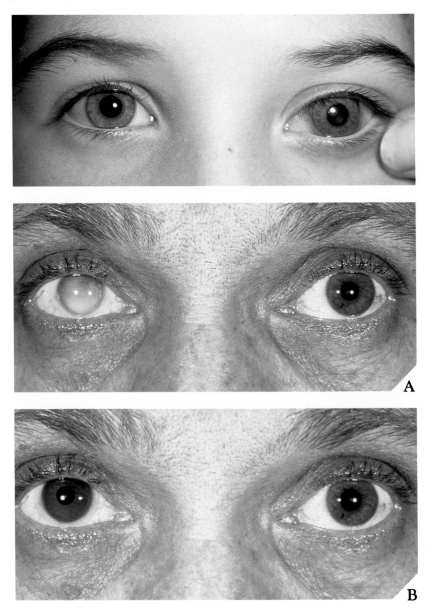

INDICATIONS FOR NONSEEING EYES

ABNORMALITIES OF THE GLOBE
Marked cosmetic improvement can be effected in an eye which is buphthalmic (Fig. 8.14).

ABNORMALITIES OF THE CORNEA
A large number of patients fitted have corneal leukomas secondary to surgical or nonsurgical trauma. A large number of leukomas are in failed corneal grafts. Another large percentage of the corneal leukomas are from congenital abnormalities (e.g., Peter's anomaly) (Fig. 8.15).

ABNORMALITIES OF THE IRIS
Eyes disfigured by occluded or secluded pupils can be improved cosmetically with these lenses.

ABNORMALITIES OF THE LENS
An easy, noninvasive method for disguising cataracts in blind eyes or in otherwise inoperable eyes is the placement of a so-called "pupil blackout" or totally opaque lens on the cornea, thus covering the disfiguring cataract (Fig. 8.16).

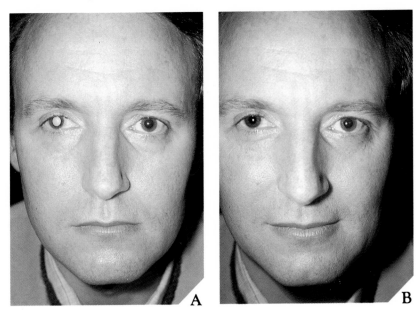

Fig. 8.16 (A) *Nonoperable cataract in right eye without contact lens.* (B) *Nonoperable cataract covered by opaque prosthetic lens.*

VITREORETINAL ABNORMALITIES

Surprisingly, a large number of patients with blind eyes experience extreme photophobia, especially if the cause of blindness is retinal detachment plus vitreal bleeding. A prosthetic lens relieves the photophobia.

INDICATIONS FOR TINTED PROSTHETIC LENSES IN SIGHTED EYES

SYSTEMIC DISORDERS

Albinotic patients with photophobia often gain great benefit from light-blocking lenses. Patients with rod monochromatism and cone dystrophy are severely photophobic. Use of the lenses for photophobia obviates the need for the use of dark goggles, which reduces visual field and makes the patient look strange (Fig. 8.17).

ABNORMALITIES OF THE CORNEA

BULLOUS KERATOPATHY In eyes with bullous keratopathy, tinted prosthetic lenses are useful, both therapeutically and cosmetically (Fig. 8.18).

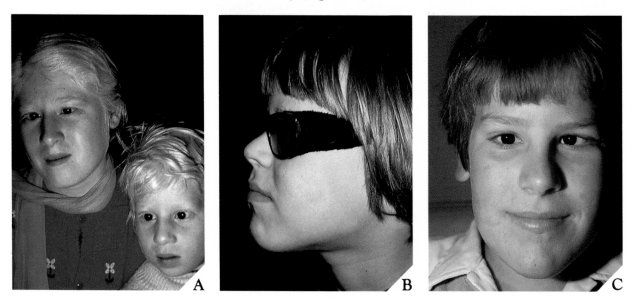

Fig. 8.17 (A) *Pakistani albinos wearing "sunshade" soft contact lenses.* (B) *Extremely photophobic monochromat wearing disfiguring goggles* which restrict the visual field. (C) *Same child as in (B), wearing deeply tinted lenses which allow for normal appearance and full physical activity.*

CHRONIC UVEITIS AND BAND KERATOPATHY In patients with chronic uveitis who develop band keratopathy, the lenses reduce photophobia and obscure the band keratopathy.

TRAUMATIC CORNEAL SCARRING These patients not only have photophobia, but also irregular astigmatism. Soft contact lenses can reduce the irregular astigmatism, and the tint reduces the photophobic symptoms from dispersion of light. The resultant astigmatism can often be corrected with a toric soft contact lens (Fig. 8.19).

KERATOREFRACTIVE SURGERY Patients who have photophobia as a result of corneal refractive surgery often benefit from tinted prosthetic lenses.

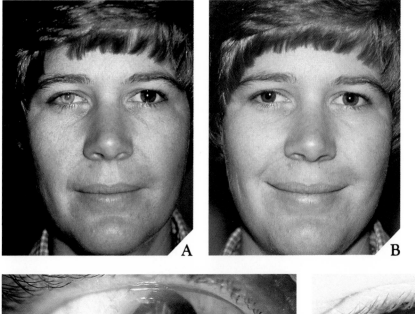

Fig. 8.18 (A) *Bullous keratopathy in right eye without contact lens.* (B) *Patient wearing cosmetic/therapeutic lens.*

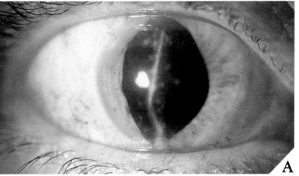
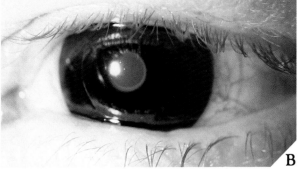

Fig. 8.19 (A) *Corneal scar and iridoplegia.* (B) *Prosthetic lens can reduce the photophobia and* *irregular astigmatism and avoids the corneal scar by decentration of the visual axis on the lens.*

HETEROCHROMIA Heterochromia can be neutralized with prosthetic lenses (Fig. 8.20).

ABNORMALITIES OF THE IRIS AND IRIDIA

Patients benefit from the use of pseudo-iris cosmetic lenses. These lenses reduce light sensitivity, and their "pinhole effect" aids vision in patients with macular aplasia (Fig. 8.21).

TRAUMATIC AND NEUROLOGIC IRIDOPLEGIA Patients with traumatic and neurologic iridoplegia not only have improvement of cosmetic appearance, but also reduction of photophobia.

LARGE COLOBOMAS OR INADVERTENT IRIDECTOMIES/IRIDOTOMIES Patients with these defects obtain relief from photophobia with tinted lenses (Fig. 8.3).

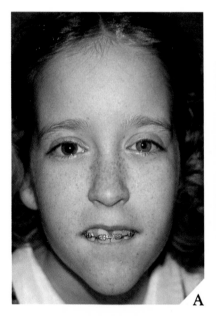
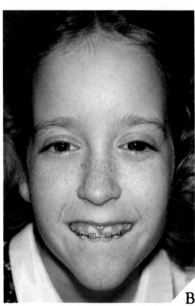
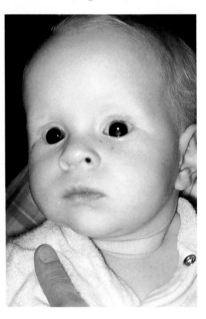

Fig. 8.20 (A) *Congenital heterochromia in patient without contact lens.* (B) *Congenital* *heterochromia in patient wearing translucent contact lens.*

Fig. 8.21 *Congenital aniridia.*

ABNORMALITIES OF THE LENS

APHAKIA AND PSEUDOPHAKIA, WITH PHOTOPHOBIA
Tinted contact lenses can reduce photophobia in patients with displaced pseudophakos. In eyes with subluxated lenses, a prism-ballasted soft contact lens can be fitted and selectively tinted to produce a clear pupillary aperture in either the aphakic or phakic portion of the visual pathway.

VITREORETINAL ABNORMALITIES
Vitreous hemorrhages are often associated with photophobia. Light-blocking lenses can alleviate this problem.

MACULOPATHY
Patients with glare symptoms can be helped with tinted lenses. The "pinhole effect" can maximize vision.

EXTRAOCULAR MUSCLE DISORDERS
Central "pupil blackout" lenses will eliminate diplopia in patients with various strabismus problems [e.g., diabetic ocular muscle palsy (temporary problem) and failed strabismus surgery (permanent problem)]. This has become a very important and widely used indication for these lenses (Fig. 8.22).

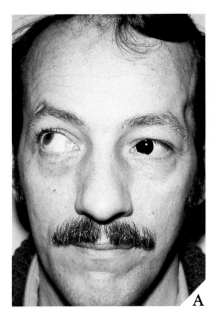

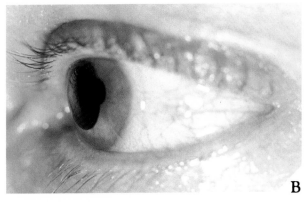

Fig. 8.22 Diplopia. (A) Third-nerve palsy cerebral aneurysm. (B) Center blackout lens stops central diplopia and preserves peripheral vision.

AMBLYOPIA

Some patients are sensitive to occluder patch wearing because of allergy or vanity. "Blackout patch" lenses have been used successfully for the treatment of amblyopia (Fig. 8.23).

COLOR BLINDNESS

Luminescence of any color can be enhanced using a lens tinted with a specific color wavelength. Red lenses have been used with varying degrees of success in deuteranopes (Fig. 8.24).

INDICATIONS FOR TINTED PROSTHETIC LENSES—SUMMARY

In summary, the most important indications for tinted prosthetic lenses are (a) improvement of cosmetic appearance, (b) reduction of photophobia, (c) maximization of visual potential, and (d) elimination of diplopia.

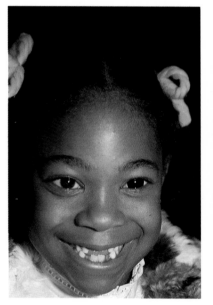

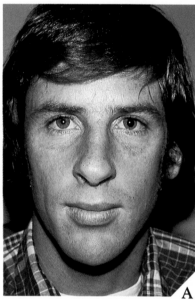

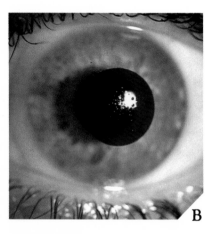

Fig. 8.24 (A) *Red-green color blindness with* (B) *red filter lens.*

Fig. 8.23 *"Blackout patch" lens for treatment of amblyopia.*

LENSES FOR EXPERIMENTATION

Tinted lenses have been used to study visual perception, extraocular muscle movements, color vision, visual deprivation, amblyopia, visual field deprivation, and vestibular ocular function. The Narcissus Foundation has provided NASA with specially marked lenses to help record exquisite eye movements for the study of the causes of space sickness. They were used in Space Lab I and IV experiments (13) (Fig. 8.25). Tinted lenses have been used to light-shield the eyes of animals in captivity whose normal habitat is dark (e.g., deep-water sharks) (Fig. 8.26).

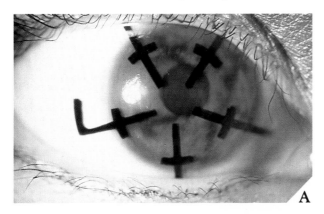

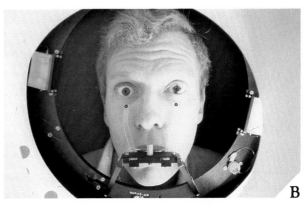

Fig. 8.25 (A) *and* (B) *NASA—Special markings on this, the first contact lens in space, facilitated* collection of eye movement data for computerized analysis in space-sickness experiments.

Fig. 8.26 *The author fitting a deep-water shark suffering from photophobia at Steinhart Aquarium, San Francisco.*

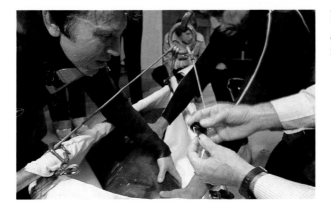

SPECIALTY LENSES

Surgical protective lenses, bifocal lenses, and sports lenses for shooting, sailing, and surfing are among the many unifunctional lenses designed around selective tinting imagery (Fig. 8.27).

FITTING TECHNIQUE

Although the technique of fitting prosthetic soft contact lenses on nondisfigured eyes is not very different from routine contact lens fitting, the problems are markedly increased when the eye has been physically damaged or has an abnormal configuration. These difficulties are usually compounded because keratometric readings cannot be obtained from such an eye. For these reasons, fitting is carried out on an individual basis with fitting sets. The initial lens is chosen on the basis of external evaluation of the eye and intuition. The lens is placed on the eye and observed for adequate covering of the defect and adequate movement in order to avoid a tight lens.

Color determination and specific imaging such as pupillary size, iris size, and specific iris details often can be incorporated with the help of color photographs of both eyes. The easiest and

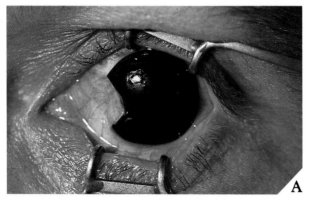
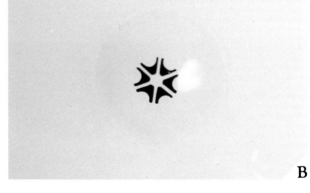

Fig. 8.27 (A) *Surgical lens protects eye from light and prevents patient from seeing procedure. Described by L. Meshel in Ref. (6). (B) Soft bi-* *focal lens design based on hard bifocal device described by Dr. George Jessen.*

most efficient method of lens design, however, is to work from trial lenses. In this way, the specific centering characteristics of the lens on the patient's eye can be determined. One can decide if displaced imagery on a prism-ballasted lens is necessary to achieve the best cosmetic results.

LENS CARE

Generally, daily surfactant cleaning and cold (chemical) disinfection are recommended.

COMPLICATIONS

Specific complications associated with cosmetic or prosthetic lenses have not occurred. Any complications are similar in type, frequency, and severity to those encountered with the routine use of soft lenses, either on a daily-wear or an extended-wear basis.

CONCLUSION

The theoretical suggestions concerning tinting made by Wichterle in the late 1950s have become clinical realities (Fig. 8.28). Soft contact lens tinting has proven to be an im-

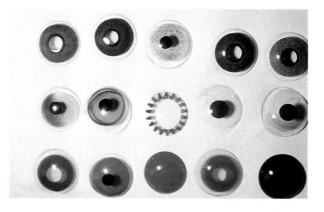

Fig. 8.28 *Tinted lenses—overview.*

portant feature for many different types of lens wearers, especially for those who require therapeutic and prosthetic lenses. There will certainly be dramatic advances in opaque lens technology, as well as in designs for fashion lenses, in the future (Fig. 8.29).

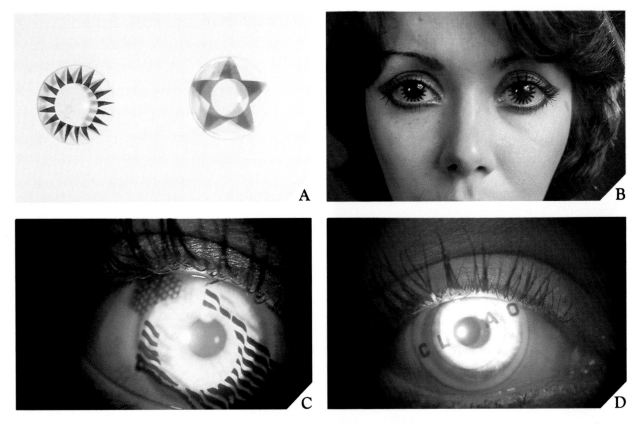

Fig. 8.29 (A) and (B) Fashion lenses of the future? (C) and (D) Advanced tinting methods allow for the reproduction of any image on any soft contact lens. This permits exquisite prosthetic imagery. (Photos from the Narcissus Medical Research Foundation.)

REFERENCES

1. Wichterle, O. Selectively light absorbing contact lenses. U.S. Patent 3,476,499, November 4, 1969.

2. Wichterle, O. Method of forming color effects in hydrogel contact lenses and ophthalmic prosthesis. U.S. Patent 3,679,504, July 25, 1972.

3. U.S. FDA approval. D & C Green 6 for use in soft contact lenses, March 1983.

4. U.S. FDA approval. Coloration for placing indices on soft contact lenses, Precision Cosmetic Co./L. G. Meshel, May 1983.

5. U.S. FDA approval. Four VAT dyes for use on soft contact lenses. Custom Tint Laboratories, September 1983.

6. Meshel, L. Second generation soft contact lenses. *Contact Intraocul. Lens Med J.*, 2:26, 1976.

7. Meshel, L. Tinted lenses: New life for dead eyes. *Contact Lens Forum*, 3:13, 1978.

8. Weinstock, Frank J. Hydrophilic lens pigmentation. *Arch. Ophthalmol.*, 91:6, 1974.

9. Knapp, J. Z. U.S. Patent, 4,582,402, April 1986.

10. Fatt, Irving, O.D., Oh.D. Personal correspondence, 1980.

11. Meshel, L. Prosthetic contact lenses. In: Dabezies, O. (Ed.), *Contact Lens Association of Ophthalmologists: The CLAO Guide to Basic Science and Clinical Practice*, Vol. II, pp. 59.1–59.8, Grune & Stratton, New York, 1984.

12. Meshel, L. Prosthetic soft contact lenses: Rehabilitation of the traumatized eye. In: Miller D. Stegmand (Ed.), *Treatment of Anterior Segment Ocular Trauma* Medicopia, Montreal, Canada, 1986.

13. Young, L. R., et al. Spatial orientation in weightlessness and readaptiation to earth's gravity. *SCI*, 225:205–208, 1984.

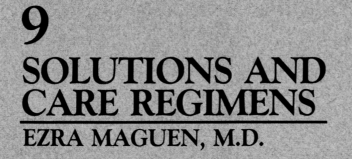

9
SOLUTIONS AND
CARE REGIMENS
EZRA MAGUEN, M.D.

Contact lens care has proven itself over time not only as a method to clean the contact lenses but also as a safety device that protects the patient wearing contact lenses. A whole array of pathological conditions related to faulty care of contact lenses has become evident over the years. Some clinical conditions such as infectious keratitis related to contact lenses may result in permanent damage to the patient's cornea as well as reduction in vision. Other conditions such as giant papillary conjunctivitis may result in the permanent inability to wear contact lenses and in significant discomfort.

In addition, the contact lens care industry has grown tremendously, and the investment of effort and money in contact lens care-related research and development is very significant.

Prior to describing the various methods of lens care, a discussion will be provided on contact lens spoilage. The types of lens solution will be enumerated, and the methods of cleaning and disinfection of hard and soft contact lenses will be discussed, and adverse reactions related to lens care will be described.

CONTACT LENS SPOILAGE

Spoilage of contact lenses has been recognized not only as a major reason for the turnover of contact lenses in certain patients but also as a major cause for ocular pathology in contact lens wearers (1–3).

The elements that contribute to contact lens deposits and spoilage, particularly in soft contact lenses, can be classified as follows:

1. Organic elements. These include: proteins (especially lysozyme); free amino acids; polysaccharides; glycoproteins; lipids; mucins; drugs; cosmetics; a variety of organic pigments; environmental pollutants; and microbial contaminants (mainly opportunistic flora of the conjunctiva and lid, as well as other bacteria and fungi).
2. Inorganic elements. These include: calcium salts (phosphates and carbonates); mercury, iron, and other metal compounds; silicon; and magnesium and sodium salts.
3. Mixed elements. These include: mucoprotein–lipid complex with or without organic and inorganic elements.
4. Manufacturing and physical defects. These include: polymer impurity; aging; and decay.

CLINICAL TECHNIQUES OF IDENTIFICATION

Contact lens spoilage in its advanced stages may be seen without optical aids by gross examination of the contact lenses. (Fig. 9.1). Earlier evidence of contact lens spoilage will need to be evaluated with the slit lamp. This instrument is indeed invaluable in determining the presence of contact lens spoilage, and examination of every contact lens patient should include slit-lamp examination of the contact lenses themselves. Direct slit-beam illumination will show such dense deposits as calcific and mixed deposits. Indirect illumination and technique comparable to "sclerotic scatter" will allow the viewing of semitransparent wide patches of proteinaceous and lipid deposits. Such indirect illumination techniques also enhance the visibility of small manufacturing defects within the lens polymer.

NATURE AND PATHOGENESIS OF CONTACT LENS SPOILAGE

ORGANIC CONSTITUENTS

Organic constituents that originate from the ocular environments mostly include: proteins (lysozyme and free amino acids) derived from tears; mucoid material derived from goblet cells; and lipids and sebaceous material derived from the meibomian glands. Exogenic organic constituents (such as cosmetics and finger contaminants) and environmental pollutants (such as nicotine) also contribute to the formation of deposits. Microbial contaminants may be also present.

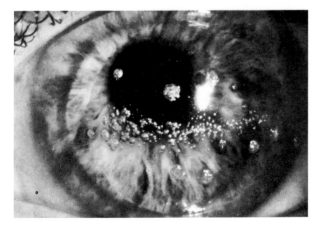

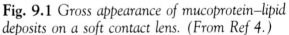

Fig. 9.1 *Gross appearance of mucoprotein–lipid deposits on a soft contact lens. (From Ref 4.)*

Proteinaceous material often deposits as a thin semiopaque or translucent superficial film that may cover the lens partially or entirely. (Fig. 9.2). Buildup of protein deposits impairs lens transparency and acuity, produces irritation and discomfort, and may lead to giant papillary conjunctivitis. The factors that favor the buildup of protein include the following: the type of polymer material; use of heat for disinfection; incomplete or reduced rate of blinking; tear deficiency; altered tear composition; and chronic allergic and giant papillary conjunctivitis.

Lipid deposits are recognizable by their greasy, smooth, shiny appearance and by fingerprint impressions. (Fig. 9.3). Such deposits often occur in combination with mucin protein as well as with calcium in its pure form.

Lipid production in the eye is increased in bacterial conjunctivitis, blepharoconjunctivitis, and meibomitis, all of which increase the incidence of lipoidal deposits. Use of certain products, such as chlorhexidine, renders the lens surface hydrophobic and lipophilic. Silicone lenses are ordinarily more lipophilic than lenses made from other material, especially when the silicone-lens surface coating has become degraded. The use of contra-

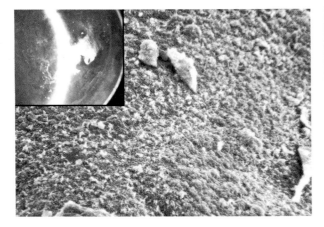

Fig. 9.2 *Proteinaceous film deposit on a soft contact lens (gross appearance) seen by scanning electron microscopy. Inset shows clinical appearance of an irregularly deposited, proteinaceous film. (Reproduced with permission from Ref. 1)*

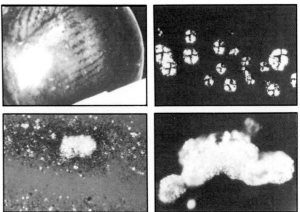

Fig. 9.3 *Lipid deposits on a soft contact lens. Top left, Greasy fingerprint impression seen grossly. Top right, Small deposits of lipid in the anterior lens matrix showing characteristic Maltese-cross pattern by polarization microscopy. Bottom left, Contamination of soft contact lens with mascara. Bottom right, Lipid deposit partly infiltrating the anterior soft lens matrix. (Reproduced with permission from Ref. 1.)*

SOLUTIONS AND CARE REGIMENS

ceptive tablets can be associated with increased lipid deposits on the lens. Lipids can be removed by detergents, anionic cleaners, and lipolytic enzymes.

Mucin deposits appear as smooth, yellowish white, opaque, filamentous or irregular jelly-like mounds (Fig. 9.4). Mucin is a common lens deposit in patients who have altered tear function of even minor conjunctival inflammation. Surface mucin can be removed by mucolytic agents and surfactant cleaners.

Pigmented deposits in soft lenses usually are related to factors such as disinfecting techniques, environmental pollutants, ocular medications, cosmetics, diagnostic agents, microbial infestations, and polymer aging. Organic pigments such as melanin- and tyrosine-like polymers appear as yellow-brown deposits just below the lens surface, often beginning from the edge of the lens. A deeply discolored lens seen against a dark background appears to have an overall blue haze and, under ultraviolet light, shows some fluorescence. Melanin-like pigmentation is common among smokers. Adrenochrome (melanin-like) pigments are deposited uniformly in soft lenses in patients using epinephrine drops for long periods of time. This problem is less common with the use of the pro-drug compound. The repeated use of eye drops containing topical vasoconstrictors such as tetrahydrozoline can cause lens discoloration. Diagnostic agents such as fluorescein and rose bengal, when left in the conjunctival sac, may stain soft lenses. High-molecular-weight fluorescein will not stain soft contact lenses. Bleaching or oxidizing agents may decolorize pigmented lenses.

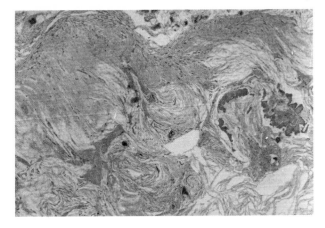

Fig. 9.4 *Mucin contamination partly infiltrating the anterior matrix of a soft contact lens. (Reproduced with permission from Ref. 1.) (Transmission electron microscopy showing mucous filaments and cellular debris.*

A heavy inoculum of bacterial organisms on a soft lens may produce a semitransparent film on the lens surface (Fig. 9.5). This is sufficient to produce symptoms of discomfort and reduced visual acuity in patients. Fungal or yeast contamination (Fig. 9.6), on the other hand, often can be recognized as a filamentous growth that can vary in color, existing in white, yellow, pink, orange-brown, and gray-black (Figs. 9.7 and 9.8). Often a fungal infestation of a lens can be correlated with the use of contaminated saline solution, water, wetting solution, or eye drops. At times, the identification of the microorganism is necessary, particularly in cases where it has produced corneal ulcers. At this point, it is important to provide the contact lenses and all contact lens cases and solution for microbiological culture examination.

INORGANIC CONSTITUENTS

The presence of protein film renders the lens surface hydrophobic. This facilitates precipitation and deposition of calcium and other inorganic deposits. Calcium salts are derived mainly from the ocular environment. Other inorganic constituents originate mostly from extraneous sources. Clinically, calcium deposits appear whitish and translucent, somewhat similar to a protein film, and may be even covered by the latter. Calcium deposits often form in the anterior, rather than posterior, surface of the lens.

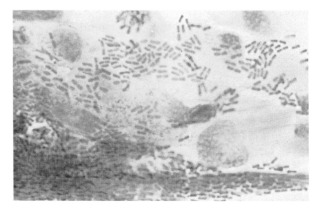

Fig. 9.5 *Semitransparent film on the surface of a soft lens results from a heavy inoculum of bacterial and fungal organisms.*

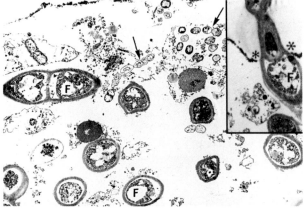

Fig. 9.6 *Microorganisms in soft contact lens matrix. Both fungal organisms (F) and bacteria (arrow) are seen in their proliferative phases. Asterisks denote lens surface through which a fungal hypha has penetrated the lens matrix (inset). (Reproduced with permission from Ref. 4.)*

(Fig. 9.9). They often are present in the interpalpebral zone. Some calcium deposits may be found within the matrix of the lens and are usually a result of loss of the structure and integrity of that lens. Factors that predispose to the formation of calcium deposits include the following: altered tear composition; low tear break-up time; dry eye syndrome; dry atmosphere; poor blinking; breakdown of lens polymer; and cleaning and disinfecting techniques. Calcium deposits in the early stages may be removed by solutions containing EDTA.

A lens with mercury deposits appears gray to grayish-black. The deposits usually arise from exogenic sources such as thimerosal-preserved saline used for disinfection. This is especially true when the lenses are heated.

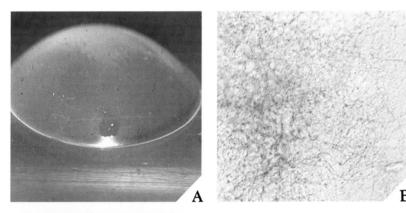

A   B

Fig. 9.7 (A) Fungal contamination on the surface of a soft lens. (B) Gross appearance of a diffuse grayish deposit on the contact lens.

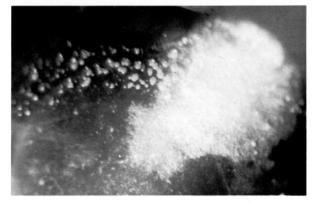

Fig. 9.8 Yeast contamination on the surface of a soft lens.

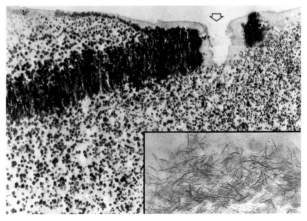

Fig. 9.9 Granular deposits of calcium in soft lens. The greatest concentration is in the area adjacent to the surface defect (arrow). Inset shows needle-shaped apatite crystals of calcium at higher magnification. (Reproduced with permission from Ref 4.)

MIXED DEPOSITS

Mixed deposits consisting of mucous, protein, and lipid (with or without calcium) are probably the most frequent cause of lens spoilage. The discrete deposits typically form raised circular or oval mounds (Fig. 9.10). They are arranged singly or in groups, with the base firmly adherent to the lens material, and, at times, partly infiltrate the lens matrix. Mixed deposits can be recognized with the same slit-lamp techniques discussed earlier. Removal of such deposits is difficult and because a discontinuation in the lens polymer is involved, they will recur even if removed.

MANUFACTURING AND POLYMER DEFECTS; AGING AND DECAY

Manufacturing defects, which may look like lens deposits, include the following: material impurity and nonhomogeneity; bubble defect; tool marks; identification marks; scratches and chips; unfinished lens surface; and foreign bodies (Fig. 9.11). Such defects are common and vary widely from one manufacturer to another, depending on the quality control system used and on the type of manufacturing process.

The types of deposits on worn soft and hard contact lenses are similar but fewer and can be removed in a much easier fashion by cleaning or polishing the lenses (5).

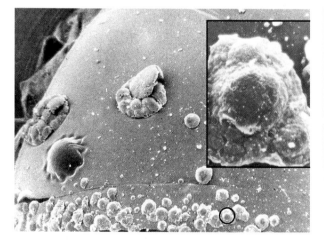

Fig. 9.10 *Mixed deposits of mucin, lipid, and protein seen on electron microscopy. Inset shows higher magnification of one deposit. (Reproduced with permission from Ref. 4.)*

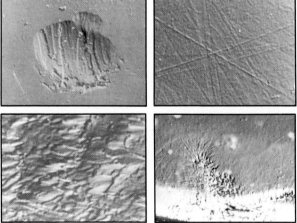

Fig. 9.11 *Surface defects in new, unworn lenses. Top left, Hemispheroidal elevation in a spin-cast lens. Top right, Diamond tool marks in a lathe cut lens. Bottom left, Rough, unpolished area. Bottom right, Edge split. (Reprinted with permission from Ref. 4.)*

CONTACT LENS SOLUTIONS: TYPES AND THEORY OF ACTION

WETTING SOLUTION

A wetting solution serves to increase the spreading or wettability of liquids on the plastic lens by temporarily converting the surface of the lens from a hydrophobic to a hydrophilic surface. This allows the tear film to uniformly spread over the surface of the lens rather than breaking up into droplets. It also coats and lubricates the lens, acting as a fluid buffer between the lens and cornea and the lens and upper lid, and prevents oil and debris from being transferred from the finger to the lens. During insertion it keeps the lens adherent to the finger. Wetting solutions are composed of the following:

1. Preservative—benzalkonium chloride or others.
2. Wetting agent—polyvinyl alcohol (PVA) or polyvinyl-N-vinylpyrrolidone (PVP).
3. Buffering system.
4. Methylcellulose or other viscous substance, which adds a cushioning effect.
5. Sodium chloride, which controls tonicity. The pH of the solution should be compatible with that of the precorneal film: 7.3–7.8.

Wetting solutions are almost exclusively used in conjunction with hard contact lens wear. Some patients tend to use saliva as a wetting solution. Even though saliva is chemically an excellent wetting agent, it always contains bacteria that significantly endanger the patients using these methods. This wetting method should be strongly discouraged.

CLEANING SOLUTIONS

Cleaning solutions are designed to remove various deposits on contact lenses resulting from normal wear. There are three distinct types of lens cleaners designed for soft contact lenses: surface-acting cleaners (surfactants), oxidative cleaners, and enzyme cleaners. Soaking solutions (see below) are generally used for hard contact lens cleaning.

SURFACE-ACTING (SURFACTANT) CLEANERS

Surfactants clean the daily accumulated residue of various proteins, lipids, and minerals off soft contact lenses by means of their ability to lower the surface tension of an oil/water interface. This is accomplished by incorporation of molecules that disperse oil droplets and surround them with polar molecules to create a hydrophilic surface and thus, by detergent action, facilitate removal of the debris. In some solutions, chelating agents are added to bind metallic ions (such as calcium) to prevent formation of such deposits. The removal of nondenatured protein is facilitated by the abrasive effect of rubbing the lens against the palm of the hand. Selected surfactant agents include the following: SoftMate (Barnes–Hind Hydrocurve), Pliagel (Coopervision Pharmaceuticals), and others.

OXIDATIVE AGENTS

Hydrogen peroxide has been used in a 3% solution for many years as a contact lens cleaner, particularly in Europe. Oxidizing agents are used for the removal of organic and inorganic debris. These agents oxidize organic or protein deposits and inorganic deposits and, in some instances, allow the mechanical disassembly of such deposits. Prior concerns about shortening the life span of lenses by using this method has not been proven. Recently, Lensept, a cleaning method using 3% hydrogen peroxide, has been introduced accompanied by a disk that is able, by catalysis, to neutralize the hydrogen peroxide, thereby allowing safe lens wear after use of this cleaning method. Because the use of oxidizing materials does not involve preservatives, the occurrence of allergic reactions associated with contact lens solution has been significantly reduced in our practice.

ENZYMATIC SOLUTIONS

Enzyme solutions are used as regular and periodic cleaning agents. They are composed of stabilized vegetable or animal papain, which acts by cleaving peptide linkages in the interior of protein molecules, thus creating low-molecular-weight soluble substances. More recent formulations include the following: animal protease, lipase, and mucinase (Amiclair-Amisol, Sarl, Paris, France) (6).

SOAKING AND DISINFECTING SOLUTIONS

Soaking solutions are primarily used with hard contact lenses. Their function is to eliminate, or reduce to tolerable levels, the amount of pathogens present on the lens. These solutions are able, to some extent, to remove deposits from the lens surface. The disinfection of soft contact lenses can be accomplished by thermal or chemical methods. Lenses may be thermally disinfected while resting in preserved or nonpreserved saline. A variety of thermal disinfecting units are available from different manufacturers. Chemical disinfection of soft contact lenses can be performed by both nonoxidative and oxidative chemical disinfectants (7). Nonoxidizing disinfectants include the following: chlorhexidine, thimerosal, and alkyl triethanolammonium chloride. Synergistic supplements to the main disinfectants may include the following: EDTA, sorbic acid, boric acid, and sodium borate.

The oxidizing disinfectants include the following: hydrogen peroxide, sodium dichloroisocyanurate, and povidone iodine. These systems require overnight storage in saline solution.

RINSING AND STORAGE SOLUTIONS

Rinsing and storage solutions are usually used in conjunction with soft contact lenses. They may be used with hard and gas-permeable contact lenses if necessary. Most of the preservatives used in disinfection solutions are present in the rinsing and storage solutions. The solutions are essentially used to rinse off the disinfecting and/or soaking solutions from the lens prior to insertion. To accommodate people who are allergic or who otherwise react to preservatives, the manufacturers have made available a range of nonpreserved saline solutions in large bottles and in one-time disposable units (Unisol, Refresh). Salt tablets are still available for waking-up saline solution. It has been my practice to discourage the use of such tablets because bacterial contamination of these solutions is very frequent. This may lead to corneal ulceration and significant loss of vision.

COMBINATION SOLUTIONS

Some manufacturers have combined the functions of two or three products into one single solution. Cleaning, soaking, and wetting solutions are available for hard lenses. Soaking and wetting solutions only are also found. Cleaning and storage solutions (Hydrocare and others) have been made available for soft lenses. The main drawback of these solutions is that they require the use of preservatives, and the disinfecting power of such solutions is usually reduced (8).

CLEANING AND DISINFECTION OF LENSES

SOFT LENSES
METHOD OF CLEANING
Soft lenses may be cleaned by four different methods, each one having advantages and disadvantages.

USING SURFACTANT CLEANING AGENTS. The single most important stage in soft contact lens cleaning is the use of surface-acting cleaners (surfactants). A drop or two of surface-acting solution such as SoftMate (Barnes–Hind Hydrocurve) or Pliagel (Coopervision Pharmaceuticals) is placed on the lens, which is held in the palm of the hand with its concave side up. The lens is rubbed lightly with the fingertip. The lens is then inverted and cleaned in the same manner. Prior to soft lens cleaning, hands should be washed to remove residues, particularly lipid residues. The use of soap without fragrance is recommended.

USING OXIDATIVE AGENTS. Oxidative agents based on hydrogen peroxide may also be used for cleaning lenses (see subsection on disinfection for a description of the cleaning method with oxidative agents).

USING ENZYME CLEANERS. Enzyme cleaners are primarily used to remove protein film from soft and gas-permeable contact lenses. The lens is placed with the cleaning tablet and distilled water in a vial which is filled as recommended. The vial is shaken until the tablet is dissolved. The lens should be left in the vial for a minimum of 2 hr but may be left in it overnight. The lens is then removed, rinsed, and disinfected by the procedure recommended by the practitioner. This adjunct to the cleaning of soft contact lenses should be practiced weekly, on the average. The frequency of use should be determined by how fast the particular patient coats his lenses with protein deposits. It should be practiced more frequently in patients who use heating disinfection methods.

USING THE ULTRASONIC CLEANING METHOD. We have found the mechanical action of ultrasound to be extremely efficient in removing some of the surface debris that accumulates on contact lenses. In addition, in those patients who react to preservatives or other chemicals, we have found that multiple passages of lenses with nonpreserved rinsing solutions through ultrasonic cleaning reduces symptoms, probably by diluting those chemicals from the interstitial spaces of the lens polymer. Lenses should be placed in rinsing solutions, preserved or nonpreserved as deemed necessary by the manufacturer, and placed in the ultrasonic cleaner for an average of 30 min. This procedure may be repeated as necessary until the contact lenses are comfortable.

DISINFECTION

HEAT DISINFECTION. The materials necessary for heat disinfection include preserved or nonpreserved rinsing solution, a contact lens case, and a contact lens heating unit. Contact lens cases and heating units are available in one package from several manufacturers. The earliest heat disinfection unit available on the market was rather cumbersome, but further developments provided smaller-size, more compact units which may be used even when the lens wearer is traveling.

The following steps are necessary to undertake heat disinfection of contact lenses:

1. The lenses are cleaned with surfactant as outlined above.
2. The lenses are rinsed well with saline solution.
3. The lenses are placed in the lens container filled with either nonpreserved or preserved saline solution.
4. The lens case is placed in the heating unit, and distilled water is added as recommended by the manufacturers. In some units, the saline solution present in the lens container is sufficient and no further fluid is necessary.
5. The unit is turned off or will turn itself off automatically when the procedure is complete. The lenses may be left in the case overnight or worn immediately. It is recommended to use a small amount of rinsing solution to reduce the lens' temperature if the patient is considering wearing the lenses immediately after boiling.

There are several advantages to this cleaning method: It is a more effective means of sterilization and it is a cheaper method for the patient. In addition, it is a safe method of disinfection in patients who are unable to use chemical preservatives because of sensitivities or allergies.

The main disadvantage of this method is that more lens deposits and a higher rate of lens replacement can be expected by using it (9). In addition, mechanical failure of the units has been previously documented whereby the switch-off mechanism does not activate and the boiler unit, case, and lenses are destroyed. In the older boiling units, the inner surface may become mineralized, which reduces the effectiveness of the units.

CHEMICAL DISINFECTION. A large variety of contact lens solutions for chemical disinfection are available, usually in the form of whole lens cleaning systems. It is always recommended to use one cleaning system rather than mix and match solutions. Chemical disinfecting systems usually include the following combinations:

1. Surfactant, storing solution, rinsing solution or
2. Cleaning and storage solution, rinsing solution or
3. Hydrogen-peroxide-operated systems.

SURFACTANT–STORAGE–RINSING SYSTEMS. The following steps are necessary for disinfection with the systems:

1. Remove the lens from the eye.
2. Place the lens in the palm of the hand, pour a few drops of surfactant cleaner on the lens, and rub gently.
3. Rinse the lens with rinsing solution.
4. Place the lens in the lens container and add storing solution until the lens is well immersed.
5. Remove the lens from the case.
6. Rinse the lens with rinsing solution, then insert into eye.
7. Empty the case, rinse it with warm tap water, and air-dry.

CLEANING-AND-STORAGE–RINSING SYSTEMS. The procedure with this system is as follows:

1. The lens is removed from the eye, placed on the palm of the hand, and cleaned with a cleaning and storage solution.

2. The lens is rinsed with the same solution and placed in the container.
3. The container is filled to two-thirds its capacity with the above solution until the lens is well immersed.
4. Before insertion the lens is rinsed with saline.
5. The lens case is rinsed with warm tap water and then air-dried.

HYDROGEN PEROXIDE SOLUTION. The system includes a hydrogen peroxide solution bottle, two containers (one of which includes a catalytic disk), and saline (preserved or nonpreserved). In addition, a lens cleaning solution, such as Pliagel, may be added to the regimen.

The method of procedure is as follows:

1. The lens is gently rubbed with a lens cleaning solution and then rinsed with saline.
2. The lens is placed on a lens holder which is placed in the first container containing hydrogen peroxide 3% (Lensept) and allowed to soak for 15 min.
3. The lens is then transferred to the second container containing preserved or nonpreserved normal saline and a catalyst (Septicon disk). This disk breaks down any peroxide into oxygen and water and is allowed to act in this fashion overnight or for a minimum of 6 hr.
4. The lens is rinsed with saline solution prior to wear.

A one-step cleaning and disinfecting method with hydrogen peroxide has been released under the brand name AO Sept. With this method, the lens is placed in a single container containing the catalytic disk and hydrogen peroxide for a minimum of 4 hr or as recommended by the manufacturer. Prior to lens wear, the lens is rinsed with preserved or nonpreserved saline as recommended.

Softcon lenses have been demonstrated not to adequately disinfect with chemical solutions and to deteriorate with boiling. The hydrogen peroxide system is most adequate for these lenses, yet surfactant cleaners should not be used and the lens should be initially rubbed with a preserved saline solution such as Lensrins.

It has been our practice to use this cleaning method, along with nonpreserved saline and Pliagel (Coopervision, San German, Puerto Rico) as a surfactant agent, for cleaning lenses in those patients who had previously reacted to contact lens solutions. We have also found that, overall, the use of such a cleaning system reduces the incidence of allergic and toxic reactions to contact lens solutions.

HARD LENSES

METHODS OF CLEANING

The cleaning and disinfection of hard contact lenses is a relatively easy technical problem because deposits usually do not adhere to the contact lens. Therefore, some household detergents may be satisfactory for lens cleaning. At the same time, their use is not recommended because some of these detergents may spoil the hard contact lens polymer. If these chemicals are not thoroughly rinsed, they may cause eye irritation and, in some cases, significant ocular damage.

The methods of cleaning hard contact lenses include mechanical rubbing, hydraulic cleansing, and ultrasonic cleansing.

Mechanical rubbing involves the use of a drop of cleansing solution on the hard contact lens and rubbing it between the thumb and index finger. This method is an efficient cleaning method, yet it may cause scratches on the surface of the lens.

Hydraulic cleansing involves the placement of the contact lens in a special perforated case immersed in the cleaning solution. The lens case permits back-and-forth pumping action of the contact lens receptable within the contact lens case, thereby cleaning residues of the lens surfaces by hydraulic action.

Ultrasonic cleansing involves the use of an ultrasound-wave-generating device in which the lens case is placed. The lens is immersed in cleaning solution inside the lens case. This is an efficient method of cleaning hard contact lenses. Recently, such devices have been available at a reasonable price, making this mode of cleaning affordable for the average hard contact lens user.

LENS SOAKING AND STORAGE

Hard contact lenses may be left in soaking solution immersed in their cases until ready to be worn. Prior to wear, contact lenses should be rinsed in commercially available saline solution. A wetting solution should be applied and then the contact lens should be placed on the cornea.

Combination solutions for wetting, soaking, and rinsing are available by different manufacturers. As is the case with soft contact lenses, the efficacy of these solutions in cleaning contact lenses is less than a single solution; also, because these solutions contain preservatives, they may predispose the patient to allergic or toxic reactions. It has been our practice not to encourage the use of combination solutions and to provide those only to patients who are potentially noncompliant.

Few contact lens practitioners advocate dry storage for hard contact lenses, arguing that wet storage promotes the growth of bacteria. It has become a consensus that wet storage of hard contact lenses is preferable because soaking solutions have proven to be efficient in bacterial growth control. In addition, a PMMA contact lens absorbs 1–2% of its own weight of liquid while being stored for 12 hr in a soaking solution. Wet-stored lenses provide better wetting of their surface, whereas dry-stored lenses increase mucous production and induce the condensation of secretion on the lens surface, thereby inducing or worsening ocular irritation (10).

GAS-PERMEABLE LENSES

The cleaning of gas-permeable contact lenses is similar to the method used for hard contact lenses. Several manufacturers have devised systems specific to gas-permeable contact lenses. These systems usually include a cleaning agent and a wetting–soaking agent. Previously, the use of benzalkonium chloride was thought to be responsible in affecting the comfort of rigid gas-permeable lenses by adhering to the lens polymer. Several studies have shown that this preservative does not, in fact, adhere to the rigid gas-permeable polymers now available in the market (11).

On the other hand, rigid gas-permeable lenses have been shown to adsorb proteinaceous material, thereby causing proteinaceous deposits on the lenses. Cleaning with enzymatic cleaners, as previously outlined, helps in eliminating such deposits (12).

CONTACT LENS CASES

A great variety of contact lens cases is available on the market. In order to avoid the tearing and loss of contact lenses, contact lens cases have to fulfill a certain number of requirements.

Contact lenses should be stored loosely inside the case because contact lenses may be broken or torn when they become stuck against a snap-on device or a snap-on cover. A contact lens case should allow total immersion of a lens within it so the contact lens can be stored wet. The case should be easy to clean and should not have areas that are difficult to reach; otherwise it may become contaminated. Contaminated contact lens cases are a major source of bacteria that may be capable of infecting a contact lens. The case should be made of plastic and should not contain any sponge rubber that may concentrate chemicals or be degraded by them.

The types of cases available on the market are as follows: simple snap-top cases (Fig. 9.12A–B); cases with "snap-on basket-like" devices that allow the fixation of a soft contact lens on a convex surface (Fig. 9.13); and cases for hard or soft contact lenses with loose-fitting basket-like devices to contain the lenses (Fig. 9.14). In addition, cases are available which allow hydraulic cleaning of hard and soft contact lenses by to-and-fro pumping movement within the case (Fig. 9.15).

The daily cleaning routines for contact lenses are summarized in Fig. 9.16.

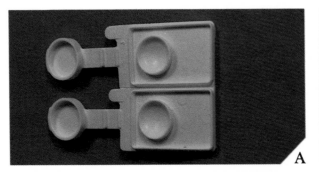
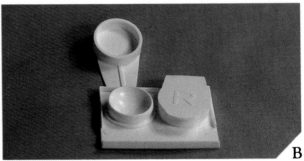

Fig. 9.12 (A) *Snap-top case for hard contact lenses.* (B) *Snap-top case for soft contact lenses.*

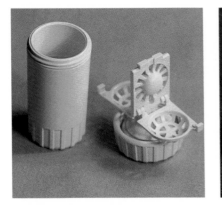
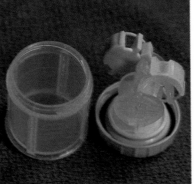
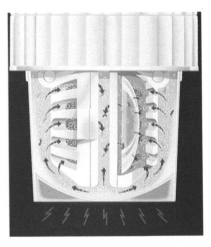

Fig. 9.13 *Contact lens case with snap-on basket-like device that allows the fixation of a soft contact lens on a convex surface.*

Fig. 9.14 *Contact lens case (for hard or soft contact lenses) with loose-fitting basket-like device to contain the lenses.*

Fig. 9.15 *Contact lens case that allows hydraulic cleaning of hard and soft contact lenses.*

ADVERSE REACTION RELATED TO CONTACT LENS CARE

CHEMICAL KERATOCONJUNCTIVITIS

Chemical keratoconjunctivitis occurs as a direct result of the chemical actions of contact lens cleaning solutions, contact lens enzyme cleaners, and hydrogen peroxide. The patient usually

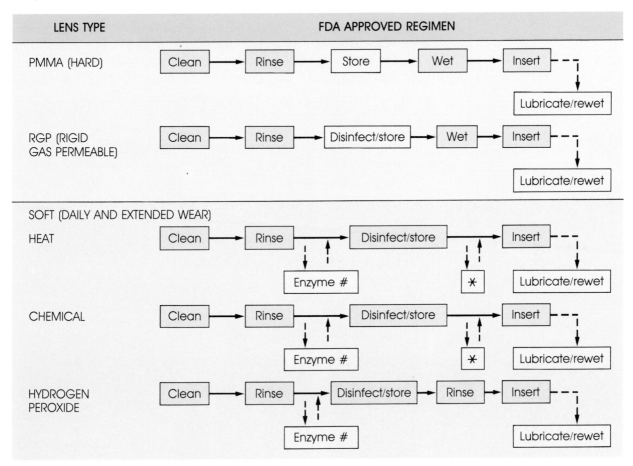

Fig. 9.16 *Summary of cleaning routines for contact lenses. The solid arrowed lines represent the daily routine or the routine recommended by your practitioner. The dashed arrowed lines include those procedures that are not necessarily routine but that are to be followed as needed or as recommended by your practitioner. The shaded boxes represent the recommended regimen to follow if routine wear is interrupted (e.g., if you must remove lens at midday because of foreign body, etc.). Note: Always wash your hands before handling your lenses and inserting them into your eyes. Asterisk refers to optional rinses; dagger refers to the fact that the use of distilled water in this procedure will not protect against contamination.*

experiences immediate discomfort upon wearing the contact lens. The patient also complains of light sensitivity and copious tearing. On slit-lamp examination, the conjunctiva is usually moderately to severely hyperemic. The cornea may show varying degrees of haze. With fluorescein, there is corneal and conjunctival punctate staining which is widespread and fairly homogeneous. Corneal epithelial defects may be seen in severe cases (Fig. 9.17). Treatment consists of immediate removal of the offending contact lens and chemical and copious rinsing of the eye with nonpreserved saline. Patching the eye for a small period of time usually may, in itself, improve this condition significantly. At the discretion of the physician, topical antibiotics or steroids may sometimes be used to relieve symptoms and inflammatory response.

The contact lens may be rinsed copiously with nonpreserved saline solution or, as an alternative, treated with repeated rinses in nonpreserved saline and repeated passages in ultrasound as previously described. If there is any question about the ability to remove the offending agent from the contact lens by diluting it, a new set of contact lenses should be prescribed.

HYPERSENSITIVITY AND ALLERGIC KERATOCONJUNCTIVITIS

Delayed hypersensitivity reactions were associated with contact lens cleaners, particularly those containing thimerosal. The onset of symptoms is usually gradual, becoming worse over a short period of time. The patients complain of increased discomfort while

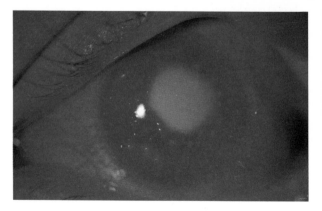

Fig. 9.17 *Corneal epithelial defect and filamentary keratopathy resulting from chemical keratoconjunctivitis.*

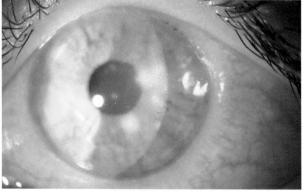

Fig. 9.18 *Subepithelial infiltrates in the cornea result from hypersensitivity to Thimerosal (Courtesy Bartly R. Mondino, MD).*

wearing contact lenses, along with redness, mucous production, and varying degrees of light sensitivity. Upon slit-lamp examination, there is a mild-to-moderate papillary response of the conjunctiva. There is a small amount of punctate staining, usually of the upper third of the cornea, and there is mild-to-moderate mucous production in the conjunctiva fornices. The cornea may show subepithelial infiltrates (13) (Fig. 9.18), stromal infiltrates (Fig. 9.19), or generalized deep corneal haze (Fig. 9.20).

Giant papillary conjunctivitis is characterized by erythema, itching under the upper lid, and contact lens intolerance, along with mucous production. Increasing evidence is available to suggest an immunological basis for this entity. The antigens that probably induce giant papillary conjunctivitis may coat soft, gas-permeable, and, more rarely, hard contact lenses (14). In addition, there is evidence that contact lens coating recurs quickly in soft contact lenses following cleaning and that contact lenses worn and cleaned regularly contain more deposits after cleaning with a surfactant or enzyme than after cleaning with a combination cleaner (15).

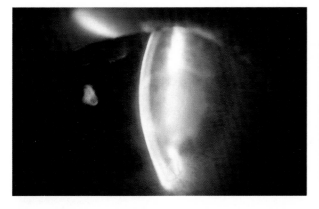

Fig. 9.19 *Stromal infiltrates in the cornea as a result from hypersensitivity to preservatives in contact lens solutions.*

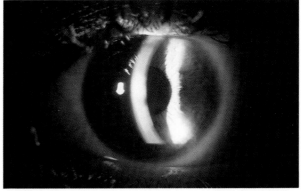

Fig. 9.20 *Generalized deep corneal haze (slitlamp view) results from hypersensitivity to preservatives in contact lens solutions.*

With slit-lamp examination, the upper tarsal conjunctiva shows characteristic papillae (Fig. 9.21), and the cornea may show superficial punctate staining on its upper third.

The treatment of giant papillary conjunctivitis is rather difficult. Changing lens brands, changing solutions, and using non-preserved solutions have only partial success. The use of sodium chromolyn, which is commercially available in its 4% solution under the brand name Optichrom (Fisons), helped control this problem in some cases (16).

INFECTIOUS KERATOCONJUNCTIVITIS

Infectious keratoconjunctivitis related to contact lens wear usually occurs because of a mechanical injury to the cornea and its invasion with bacteria. The bacteria may be present in the con-

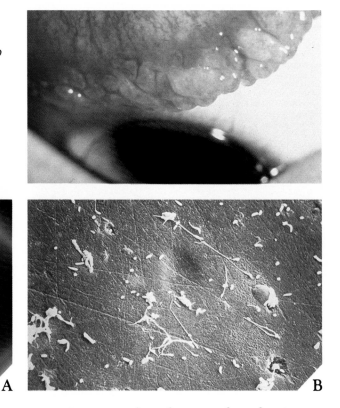

Fig. 9.21 *Characteristic papillae in the upper tarsal conjunctiva results from hypersensitivity and keratoconjunctivitis, as seen during slit-lamp examination.*

Fig. 9.22 (A) Pseudomonas, *the most common most virulent bacterium causing corneal ulcers related to contact lens wear.* (B) *Scanning elec-* tron microscopy of a soft contact lens showing adhesion of Pseudomonas *to its surface.*

junctival cul-de-sacs or may adhere to the soft contact lens. An additional source of bacterial and fungal contamination is contaminated nonpreserved saline (17–19). The symptoms may vary in severity. The onset may be gradual or acute and consists of moderate-to-severe pain, redness, light sensitivity, and purulent discharge. Slit-lamp examination reveals follicular conjunctival response, with varying degrees of mucopurulent discharge. The findings on the cornea may include localized surface haze, a central or peripheral infiltrate of varying sizes, and, in the worst case, corneal ulceration. Many pathogens may cause corneal ulceration. Pseudomonas appears to be the most common and most virulent bacterium causing corneal ulcers (Fig. 9.22A). Pseudomonas has been shown to adhere to contact lenses (Fig. 9.22B) making this organism more resistant to many of the cleaning regimens. Recently, Acanthamoeba species that are resistant to treatment have been identified as causing corneal ulceration, which may result in the loss of the eye (Fig. 9.23A and B).

The diagnosis of a corneal ulcer constitutes an emergency. Cultures should be taken from the conjunctiva, lids, and cornea. The cornea should be scraped, and the product of scraping should be placed directly into culture plates. Aggressive antibiotic treatment should be instituted prior to obtaining the results of the culture, and the contact lens should be removed immediately. The contact lens, as well as the swabs from the contact lens case and solutions, should be placed in culture to help identify

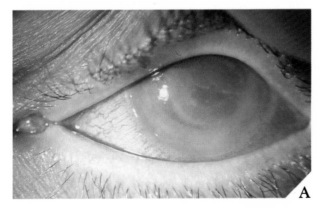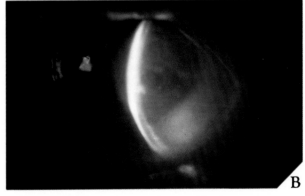

Fig. 9.23 (A) Corneal ulceration caused by Acanthameba species (external view). Note the characteristic dense peripheral ring. (B) Corneal ulceration caused by Acanthameba species (slit-lamp view).

the offending organism (Fig. 9.24). If a decision is made to resume the wearing of contact lenses following the resolution of infectious keratoconjunctivitis, the soft contact lenses should be discarded and a new pair should be provided. The fit of hard or soft contact lenses should be thoroughly reevaluated and corrected if necessary.

PREVENTION OF COMPLICATIONS

Every contact lens fitter, particularly those who fit lenses for extended wear, should undertake a few preventive measures to avoid serious ocular complications.

The importance of compliance with a prescribed cleaning regimen should be stressed to the patient. It is extremely important to ensure that patients understand fully the cleaning regimen for their lenses, that no patient should walk out of the fitter's office without the fitter having ascertained that the patient fully understood the cleaning regimen.

In addition, it is important to stress to patients that they should not use any generic solutions, unless such are approved by the fitter, since generic solutions may be incompatible with other solutions or with the type of lens the patient wears. Additionally, some cleaning materials, such as salt tablets and homemade saline solution, may put patients at higher risk of serious complications. It has been our practice to firmly discourage the use of such solutions.

Patients should be reminded that when symptoms occur with contact lens wear, the lens should be removed immediately. If removing the lens does not help, the patient should notify and see the fitter immediately. It has been our practice to provide the patient with written material on lens handling and cleaning. It is felt that this type of material not only clarifies to the patient

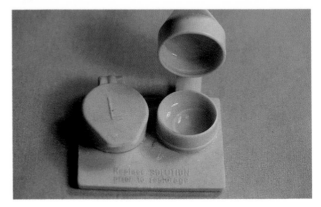

Fig. 9.24 *Soiled soft contact lens case belonging to a patient who presented with a corneal ulcer.* Pseudomonas *was cultured from both contact lens and contact lens case.*

his/her regimen after he/she has left the office but also makes the patient feel more committed to such a regimen. In addition, it has been our practice to have patients sign informed consent forms for extended-wear lenses. Copies of such informed consent may be obtained through the Contact Lens Association of Ophthalmologists and it is suggested that local legal council approve the use of the CLAO informed consent wording.

ACKNOWLEDGMENTS

This work has been supported by the Discovery Fund for Eye Research and by the National Keratoconus Foundation, Los Angeles, California.

I wish to thank Ramesh C. Tripathi MD, Ph.D whose contributions to this chapter are invaluable.

REFERENCES

1. Tripathi, R. C., and Tripathi, B. J. Soft lens spoilage: Nature, etiology and pathogenesis. *Ophthalmic Forum,* 2(2):80–91, 1984.

2. Tripathi, R. C. Soft lens spoilage. In: M. Ruben, (Ed.), *Soft Contact Lens Chemical and Applied Technology,* John Wiley & Sons, New York, 1978.

3. Maguen, E. M., et al. A long term evaluation of myopic extended wear lenses in a primary care non-referral population. *CLAO J.* (in press).

4. Tripathi, R. C., Tripathi, B. J., and Ruben, M. The pathology of soft contact lens spoilage. *Ophthalmology,* 87:365–380, 1980.

5. Fowler, S. A., Korb, D. R., Finnemore, V. M., and Allansmith, M. R. Surface deposits on worn hard contact lenses. *Arch. Ophthalmol.,* 102:757–759, 1984.

6. Josephson, J., et al. Hydrogel lens solutions. *Int. Ophthalmol. Clin.,* 21(2):163–171, 1981.

7. Rubo, S. D., and Gardner, J. F. *A Review of Sterilization and Disinfection,* Year Book Medical Publishers, Chicago, 1969.

8. Stein, H. A., and Slalt, B. J. *Fitting Guide for Hard and Soft Contact Lenses: A Practical Approach,* p. 204, C. V. Mosby, St. Louis, 1977.

9. Stein, J. M., Stark, R. L., and Randeri, K. Comparison of chemical and thermal disinfection regimens: A retrospective data analysis. *Int. Eyecare,* 2(11):570–578, 1986.

10. Hoffman, W. C. Ending the BAK–RGP controversy. *Int. Contact Lens Clin.,* 14(1):31–34, 1987.

11. Wong, M. P., Dziabo, A. J., and Kiral, R. M. Adsorption of benzalkonium chloride by RGP lenses. *Contact Lens Forum*, May:25–32, 1986.

12. Rosenthal, P., Chou, M. H., Salamone, J. C., and Israel, S. C. Protein adsorption properties of model RGP contact lens material. Presented at the CLAO meeting, Vol. 11, 1987.

13. Mondino, B. J., and Groden, L. R. Conjunctival hyperemia and corneal infiltrates with chemically disinfected soft contact lenses. *Arch. Ophthalmol.*, 98:1767–1770, 1980.

14. Fowler, S. A., and Allansmith, M. R. Evolution of soft contact lens coatings. *Arch. Ophthalmol.*, 98:95–99, 1980.

15. Fowler, S. A., and Allansmith, M. R. The effect of cleaning soft contact lenses: A scanning electron microscopic study. *Arch. Ophthalmol.*, 99:1382–1386, 1981.

16. Donshik, P. C., Ballow, M., Luistro, A., and Smartino, L. Treatment of contact lens-induced giant papillary conjunctivitis. *CLAO J.*, 10(4):346–350, 1984.

17. Smolin, G., Okumoto, M., and Nozik, R. A. The microbial flora in extended-wear soft contact lens wearers. *Am. J. Ophthalmol.*, 88:543–547, 1979.

18. Nesburn, A. B., and Maguen, E. Cosmetic lenses. *Int. Ophthalmol. Clin.*, 21(2):212–213, 1981.

19. Chalupa, E., Swarbrick, H. A., Holden, B. A., and Sjostrand, J. Severe corneal infections associated with contact lens wear. *Ophthalmology*, 94(1):17–22, 1987.

10
GIANT PAPILLARY CONJUNCTIVITIS

PETER C. DONSHIK, M.D., F.A.C.S.,
ANGELA E. LUISTRO, C.O.T., F.C.L.S.A.,
MARK BALLOW, M.D.

Clinically, the signs and symptoms can be divided into four classes (Table 10.1), starting with preclinical (in which the patient has early symptoms with minimal signs) and advancing to class 4 (in which the papillary reaction is large, with evidence of fibrovascular changes, apical staining, severe mucous produc-

TABLE 10.1
SIGNS AND SYMPTOMS OF GPC

Severity	Papillary Reaction	Mucous Production	Contact Lens Intolerance	Vision with Contact Lenses
Preclinical	Fine papillary reaction	Mild to minimal		Good vision
Mild	Papules 0.33–0.50 mm in size; minimal tarsal injection	Mild	Increased lens awareness	Good vision
Moderate	Papules 0.50 mm or larger, with elevation; beginning of subconjunctival scarring; mild tarsal injection	Moderate	Lens uncomfortable; may have excessive movement	Intermittent blurred vision
Severe	Papules 0.75 mm or larger; elevated subconjunctival scarring and apical staining tarsal injection	Moderate to severe	Lens very uncomfortable and unable to wear for any length of time	Blurred vision (depends on lens coating)

tion, conjunctival injection, punctate corneal staining, and severe contact lens intolerance) (2). Figure 10.4 shows the effects of early GPC on the tarsal plate. Figure 10.5 demonstrates the further changes associated with moderate GPC. The papules and papillary reactions characteristic of moderately advanced GPC

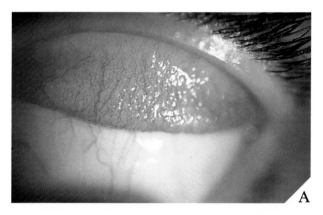

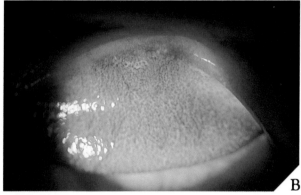

Fig. 10.4 *Early GPC. (A) Diffuse photograph of upper lid showing erythema of tarsal plate. (B) Cobalt photograph (after instillation of 2%* *fluorescein) showing diffuse papillary reaction involving all three zones of the upper tarsal plate.*

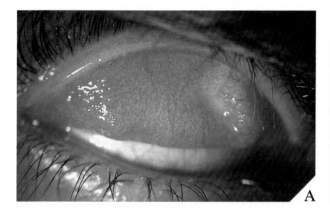

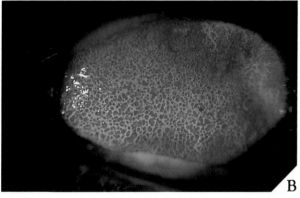

Fig. 10.5 *Moderate GPC. (A) Diffuse photograph showing erythema of upper tarsal plate. The appearance is more congested than in Fig. 10.1. (B) Cobalt photograph (after instillation of 2% fluorescein) showing larger (0.25–0.50 mm)* *papillary reaction. The papules are more clearly defined, and all three zones are involved. The majority of the larger papules (0.50 mm) are found in zones 2 and 3.*

are presented in Figs. 10.6 and 10.7. Increasing papillary reactions and subconjunctival scarring are shown in Figs. 10.8 and 10.9, which illustrate advanced GPC. The symptom complex can be associated with ocular prosthesis (9), sutures following cataract extraction (10–12) (Figs. 10.10 and 10.11), and reactions following corneal transplant surgery (13).

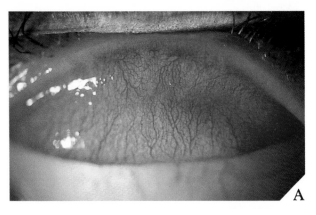

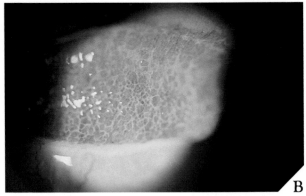

Fig. 10.6. *Moderately advanced GPC. (A) Diffuse photograph showing mild injection of the tarsal plate, with the papules being more readily visualized with white light. (B) Cobalt photo-* *graph (after the instillation of 2% fluorescein) showing large papules (0.75–1 mm) involving predominantly zones 2 and 3. The papillary reaction in zone 1 is approximately 0.50 mm in size.*

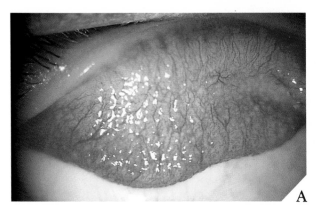

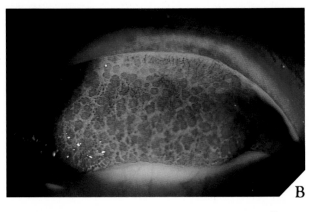

Fig. 10.7 *Moderately advanced GPC. (A) Papillary reaction is more easily visualized in the diffuse white light photographs. (B) Large, pap-* *ules (1 mm) well-defined in size involving all three zones.*

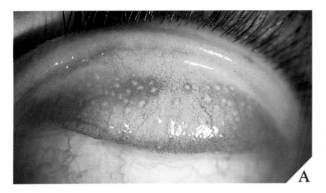

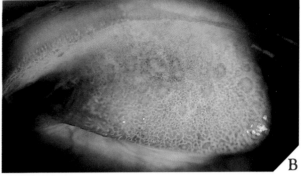

Fig. 10.8 *Advanced GPC. (A) Diffuse photograph showing papillary reactions in zone 2 which are elevated and have a whitish appearance to them. (B) Cobalt photograph (after the* instillation of 2% fluorescein) showing a large papillary reaction in the presence of a generalized papillary reaction of all three zones.

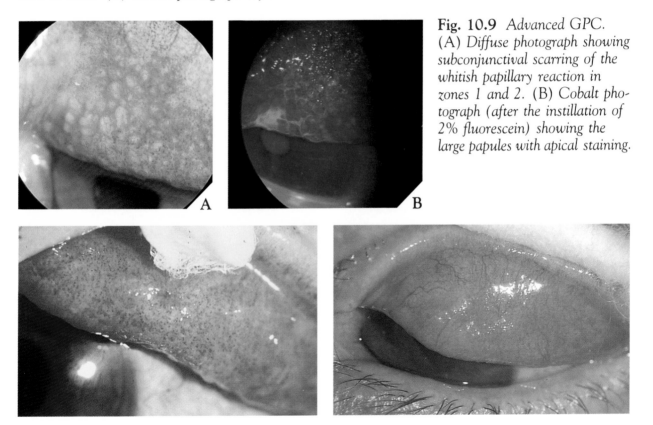

Fig. 10.9 *Advanced GPC. (A) Diffuse photograph showing subconjunctival scarring of the whitish papillary reaction in zones 1 and 2. (B) Cobalt photograph (after the instillation of 2% fluorescein) showing the large papules with apical staining.*

Fig. 10.10 *Upper tarsal conjunctiva showing papillary reaction in patient following cataract extraction. Papillary reaction is due to exposed 10-0 nylon sutures.*

Fig. 10.11 *Upper tarsal conjunctiva showing resolution of papillary reaction 3 weeks after the sutures were removed.*

INCIDENCE

The incidence of GPC is not known but is estimated to occur in approximately 10% of contact lens wearers. A study by Korb et al. (14) revealed that 10.5% of asymptomatic hard contact lens wearers had papules larger than 0.3 mm, as compared to 0.6% of noncontact lens wearers. Although asymptomatic, 76% of these patients with papillary changes in the tarsal conjunctiva had some problems associated with mucous secretion or ocular itching. However, if the patients did not have a significant papillary reaction (papules smaller than 0.3 mm), then only 8% complained of some problems associated with mucous secretion. In reviewing 150 extended-wear patients in our study, we found that 7% developed GPC. Half of the patients who developed GPC were unable to continue wearing their lenses. If one examines the upper tarsal plate of patients wearing contact lenses, it is not uncommon that a majority of patients, although asymptomatic, will have a fine papillary reaction (papules ranging in

TABLE 10.2 HISTOLOGICAL FEATURES OF UPPER TARSAL CONJUNCTIVA	
NORMAL	
EPITHELIUM:	Neutrophils Lymphocytes
SUBSTANTIA PROPRIA:	Neutrophils Lymphocytes Plasma cells Mast cells
GPC	
EPITHELIUM:	Neutrophils Lymphocytes Mast cells Eosinophils Basophils
SUBSTANTIA PROPRIA:	Eosinophils Basophils Neutrophils Mast cells Plasma cells (five classes)

size from >0.25 to <0.33 mm). Although this reaction may be due to the trauma of the contact lens against the upper lid, it is also possible that this papillary reaction may be the initial process in a chain reaction that will ultimately develop into the symptom complex that we see clinically as GPC.

HISTOLOGY

Histologically, the normal epithelium of the upper tarsal contains neutrophils and lymphocytes. Neutrophils, lymphocytes, plasma cells, and mast cells are also found in the substantia propria (15). Thus, there are no eosinophils or basophils present in the normal conjunctiva, and any mast cells that are present are limited to the substantia propria. In asymptomatic contact lens patients the conjunctival histological pattern is similar to that of a person who does not wear contact lenses (16). However, in GPC, one can identify one of the following: mast cells in the epithelium; eosinophils in the epithelium and substantia propria; and/or basophils in the epithelium and substantia propria (17) (Table 10.2). The presence of these cells (i.e, eosinophils, basophils, and mast cells) suggests an immunological process associated with the development of the signs and symptoms of GPC. This is further supported by the similarity in biopsy specimens comparing the histological appearance of the tarsal conjunctiva of patients with GPC and those with vernal conjunctivitis, a known immunologically mediated disease (18). Furthermore, plasma cells containing all five classes of immunoglobulins have been shown to be present in the substantia propria of GPC induced by prosthesis (9), and Russell bodies have been found to be present in the cytoplasma of biopsy specimens of patients with GPC (19). Thus, there is strong histological evidence that supports an immunological process mediating the pathogenesis of GPC.

TEAR ABNORMALITIES

Normal tears contain a variety of proteins that serve different physiological purposes. From the perspective of immune function, the following are of primary interest: tear immunoglobulins; components of the complement system; lactoferrin; and lysozymes. Normal values of these proteins are listed in Table 10.3. Asymptomatic contact lens wearers have normal values of these proteins. However, in patients with GPC the various tear protein components are altered. One can find elevated IgE, IgG, and IgM (Table 10.3). The elevated levels of these immunoglobulins parallel the symptomatology. When the patients are most symptomatic, the values are high. After the removal of the contact lens, as well as after the abatement of the GPC symptoms,

TABLE 10.3
TEAR IMMUNOGLOBULIN LEVELS[a]

	IgE IU/ml	IgA (mg/dl)	IgG (mg/dl)	IgM (mg/dl)
NORMAL				
Mean	1.1	16.6	1.0	<0.47
Range	0.25–1.4	7.6–36.6	0.26–3.9	0–0.47
GPC				
Mean	6.9[a]	17.0	5.1	0.3
Range	2.0–24.2	7.9–36.6	1.9–13.8	0.7–1.34

[a]Data taken from Ref. 20.

TABLE 10.4
TEAR LEVELS OF COMPLEMENT PROTEINS[a]
(AVERAGE LEVELS)

	C_3 (ng/nl)	Factor B (ng/nl)	C_3a (C_3 anaphylatoxin)
Normal	<0.3	<0.041	0
Control contact lens wearers	4.5	0.63 + 0.07	0
GPC active	17.3	2.2 + 0.6[b]	111
GPC inactive	4.5	2.2 + 0.8	0.11

[a]Data taken from Ref. 21.

immunoglobulin levels return toward normal levels. We have determined that these elevated immunoglobulin levels are locally produced by the external eye in response to a given antigen stimulus (20). Table 10.4 illustrates the elevated levels of components of the complement system—namely, C3, Factor B, and C3a (C3 anaphylatoxin)—in the tears of patients with GPC (21). Asymptomatic contact lens wearers have levels similar to those of individuals who do not wear contact lenses. The elevated complement factors are also locally produced by the external eye. Lactoferrin, a potent inhibitor of the complement system, has been shown to be significantly decreased in tears of symptomatic GPC patients (22). Lactoferrin and lysozyme are secreted by the lacrimal gland and are often used as markers for a lacrimal gland dysfunction. Thus, finding a decreased lactoferrin level could suggest the possibility of lacrimal gland dysfunction. However, we have found that while lactoferrin levels are decreased in the tears, the lysozyme levels are normal in patients who wear contact lenses as well as in those contact lens patients who develop GPC (23) (Table 10.5). Thus, the normal levels of tear lysozyme in the presence of decreased levels of lactoferrin rule out lacrimal gland dysfunction as a possible etiological factor in this syndrome complex. However, the decreased lactoferrin is an important factor in the immunopathological process occurring in GPC.

TABLE 10.5
TEAR LACTOFERRIN AND LYSOZYME LEVELS[a]
(AVERAGE LEVELS)

	Lactoferrin (mg/nl)	Total Protein (g/2)	Ratio of L/TP	Lysozyme
Normal	1.73 + 4.6	7.07 + 1.1	0.26 + 0.08	3.23 + 0.40
Contact lens control	1.57 + 0.92	7.2 + 2.2	0.25 + 1.1	3.06 + 0.70
GPC active	0.876 + 0.42	8.3 + 3.9	0.13 + 0.06	3.63 + 0.35
GPC inactive	1.33 + 0.49	6.97 + 5.9	0.26 + 0.16	5.21 + 0.86

[a]Data taken from Refs. 22 and 23.

LENS COATING

A consistent feature of this syndrome in both rigid and soft contact lens wearers is the presence of deposits coating the lens surface. The deposits can vary, ranging from a mild film (Fig. 10.12) to a heavy film with hard calcium-like deposits (Fig. 10.13). Scanning electron-microscopic studies show a variety of morphological patterns associated with the coated GPC lens (24). However, there is no obvious difference, morphologically or biochemically, between the coated lenses of patients with GPC and those of patients who do not have GPC. Soft contact lenses begin to coat after a few hours of wear. As the lens continues to be worn, more and more mucus and proteins will accumulate on the lens. The use of surfactant alone, or of enzyme cleaner alone, results in removing only 30–40% of the deposits from the lens. However, the combination of surfactant and enzyme was able to remove 75% of the deposits (25). This is strong support for the need of both cleaning modalities in removing the coated material from soft contact lenses. Because all patients with GPC have coated lenses but not all coated lenses will cause GPC, there must be either an "antigenic" difference on the coated lens or a difference in individual susceptibility. Preliminary studies (26) in our laboratory have shown some antigenic differences on coated contact lenses. The coated lenses from GPC individuals inserted into the eyes of monkeys resulted in initial elevation of tear IgE. Histopathological examinations of the upper tarsal conjunctiva showed an intense round-cell infiltrate of plasma cells and mast cells. Neither the elevated IgE

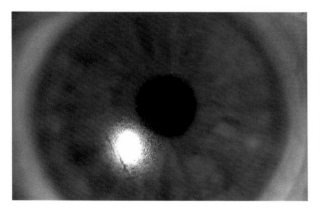

Fig. 10.12 *Mild contact lens coating in patient with GPC.*

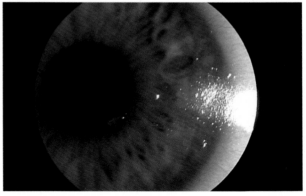

Fig. 10.13 *Hard calcium-like deposits on contact lens.*

nor the histological pattern was seen with other types of contact lenses that were inserted into monkey eyes. This further suggests that there is an antigenic material on the coated lens of GPC patients.

PATHOGENESIS

The tear immunological studies, in addition to the histopathology, strongly support an immunologically mediated basis for GPC. However, mechanical trauma has to be considered a possible contributing factor, especially in view of the presence of abnormal lid changes in over 10% of asymptomatic contact lens wearers (14). The factors that may influence mechanical trauma could be related to the diameter of the lens, the edge design of the lens, and the type of plastic used to manufacture the lens. Because the contact lens itself is probably not antigenic (normal tear immunoglobulins and histopathology in asymptomatic contact lens wearers), something must happen to the contact lens, once it is placed in the eye, to make it an "antigenic" stimulus. The most likely explanation for this antigenic change is the "coating" that occurs in the daily wearing of the lens.

Factors that can influence lens coating are: the plastic polymer of the lens, the lens design, the lens fit, and the nature of the tear secretions. Furthermore, GPC appears to be more common in the cosmetic-lens-wearing population (which is also associated with younger age groups) than in the older, aphakic population. The immunological reactivity of the external eye may be a factor in this observation. Thus, a possible hypothesis is that the mechanical trauma of the contact lens against the upper tarsal conjunctiva causes certain anatomical changes that allow the antigen which is present on the coated contact lens to be recognized, allowing an immune reaction to develop. The production of the immunoglobulins IgG and IgE (and, in the more severe cases, IgM) occurs; in addition, the complement system is activated, especially C3a. The immunological reaction attracts basophils, eosinophils, and mast cells. Both IgE and C3a can cause basophil and mast cell degranulation, releasing the active vasoamines that are responsible for the signs and symptoms of GPC (Fig. 10.14).

MANAGEMENT

The treatment of GPC which can lead to a cure is the removal of the offending stimulus—namely, having the patient discontinue wearing the contact lenses. However, most contact lens patients will not adhere to such a treatment regimen. They want to be able to continue wearing their lenses, and they seek our expertise in achieving this goal. Thus, as clinicians, we are faced with the task of trying to keep these patients happy by enabling them to continue wearing their contact lenses. Therapy can thus be directed at either keeping the antigen from developing on the lens or, once the immunological reaction has occurred, trying to modify the reaction with drug therapy.

In an attempt to alter or deter the development of the "antigen" formation on the contact lens, one can change the lens polymer, water content, diameter, or edge design. We have shown (27) that 65% of GPC patients who were refitted to a new lens identical in all parameters to the old lens were able to satisfactorily wear their lenses for an average of over 15 months. When the lens parameters were changed in some manner (e.g., the fitting was to a new but different type of lens), we observed that 77% of the patients were free of any significant symptoms or signs and were able to satisfactorily wear

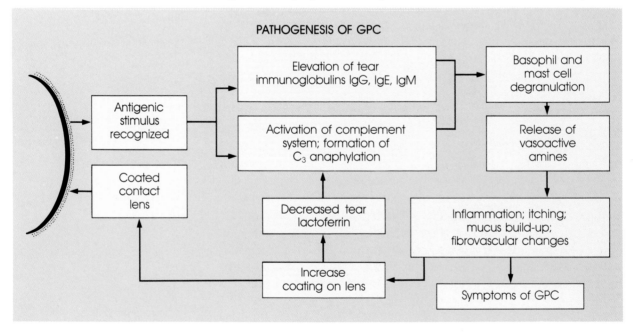

Fig. 10.14 *Pathogenesis of GPC.*

their lenses for over 11 months.

To investigate the effect of changing the lens polymer, we refitted 12 patients (23 eyes) to a new hydroxyethyl methacrylate (HEMA) lens (of a different brand): 69% of the patients were able to wear their lenses for an average of 1.4 years. When we fitted GPC patients who were wearing HEMA lenses to lenses of a different polymer (e.g., glyceryl methyl methacrylate), we observed that 79.5% were able to wear their lenses for an average of 1.6 years without difficulties.

In both groups, the failures occurred during the first 3 months after the wearer was refitted to a new lens. A significant number of a small group of patients who were changed from a rigid lens to a soft lens or from a soft lens to a rigid lens was also able to wear their lenses without a return of symptoms.

Thus, by changing the lens polymer as well as the lens design, one can successfully refit a significant number of patients who were previously symptomatic in contact lenses, without a return of their symptoms.

Therapy can also be directed at modifying the immune response. Cromolyn is a mast-cell stabilizer that will inhibit the release of vasoactive mediators from mast cells (28). Cromolyn has been shown to be effective in the treatment of allergic conjunctivitis (29,30), vernal conjunctivitis (30,31), and GPC (32). In patients who have had a return of symptoms after being refitted to a new and different lens, we have shown that the addition of cromolyn eye drops four times a day enabled 78% (7 of 9 patients) to wear their lenses without a return of symptoms (27).

Thus, on the basis of our studies, our recommendations for the management of GPC patients who want to return to lenses are as follows:

1. Have patients discontinue wearing their lenses for a minimum of 4 weeks. This allows the inflammatory process to resolve, as is evident by the resolution of symptoms and the return of abnormal tear immunoglobulins to normal levels. Patients should be free of conjunctival injection, excessive mucous secretion, and corneal punctate staining before being fitted with new lenses. The papillary reaction of the upper tarsal conjunctival surface will not change during this period. It takes months for resolution of the papules in patients who discontinue wearing lenses.

2. Refit the patient with a new (and, if possible, a different type) contact lens. If possible, we try and change the lens polymer during the refitting of the contact lens.

3. Instruct the patient on the need for meticulous care of their lenses. Patients should clean their lenses each day with a surfactant cleaner and treat their lenses with enzyme once or twice a week. We recommend that patients use nonpreserved chemicals to clean and disinfect their lenses. We feel that this helps decrease the possible sensitivity in eyes in which the immune system is already actively stimulated. It is our impression that disinfection of lenses with hydrogen peroxide system may offer some benefit in decreasing lens coating.

4. Contact lenses should be changed at the first sign of any significant coating or increased mucous secretion.

5. Patients who continue to be symptomatic following the above recommendations can be treated with sodium cromolyn eye drops. It has been our experience that cromolyn, when indicated, is only effective once the eye is free of inflammation. Thus, the patient should discontinue wearing the lens and be refitted with a new lens and, at that point, initiate sodium cromolyn eye drops four times a day. The drops should be continued for at least 3 months and then can be tapered, depending on the return of clinical symptoms (see Fig. 10.1). It is our experience that steroid drops are rarely, if ever, indicated. If there is significant inflammation, then a short course (2–3 days) may be required to treat the active inflammation. However, long-term steroid drops for the treatment of the papillary reaction is not indicated and has no effect in our experience on their resolution. Table 10.6 summarizes the management of GPC.

Although GPC can be "cured" by discontinuing the patient's use of contact lenses, we found that by following the above-mentioned regimen we could enable over 80% of our GPC patients to continue wearing contact lenses.

TABLE 10.6
MANAGEMENT OF GPC

1. Discontinue wearing lenses for 4 weeks.
2. Refit with new [and, if possible, different type (polymer)] contact lens.
3. Meticulous lens care:
   a. Nonpreserved saline;
   b. Daily cleaning;
   c. Hydrogen peroxide disinfection;
   d. Enzymatic (Papine) one to two times per week.
4. Change lens at first sign of lens coating or increased mucous secretion.
5. Add sodium cromolyn eye drops if symptoms continue. Start patient on sodium cromolyn when eye is free of inflammation and a new lens is dispensed.

REFERENCES

1. Spring, T. F. Reactions to hydrophilic lenses. *Med. J. Aust.*, 1:449–450, 1974.

2. Allansmith, M. R., Korb, D. R., Grenier, J. V., et al. Giant papillary conjunctivitis in contact lens wearers. *Am. J. Ophthalmol.*, 83:697–708, 1977.

3. Richmond, P. P., and Allansmith, M. R. Giant papillary conjunctivitis. *Int. Ophthalmol. Clin.*, 65–84, 1981.

4. Greiner, J. V., Fowler, S. A., and Allansmith, M. R. Giant papillary conjunctivitis in contact lenses. In: Dabezies, O. H. (Ed.), *CLAO Guide to Basic Science and Clinical Practice*, Vol. 2, Chapter 43, pp. 1–13, Grune and Stratton, New York.

5. Udell, I. J., and Meisler, D. M. Giant papillary conjunctivitis. *Int. Ophthalmol. Clin.*, 26:35–42, 1986.

6. Sheldon, L., Beidnew, B., Geltman, C., et al. Giant papillary conjunctivitis and ptosis in a contact lens wearer. *J. Pediatr. Ophthalmol. Strabismus*, 16(2):136–137, 1979.

7. Ferman, R. A. Bloody tears. *Am. J. Ophthalmol.*, 93:524–525, 1982.

8. Meisler, D. M., Zaret, C. R., Stock, E. L., et al. Trantas dots and limbal inflammation associated with soft contact lens wear. *Am. J. Ophthalmol.*, 89:66–69, 1980.

9. Meisler, D. M., Krachmer, J. H., and Goeken, J. A. An immunopathologic study of giant papillary conjunctivitis associated with an ocular prosthesis. *Am. J. Ophthalmol.*, 92:368–371, 1981.

10. Nirankari, V. S., Koresh, J. W., and Richards, R. D. Complications of exposed monofilament sutures. *Am. J. Ophthalmol.*, 95:515–519, 1983.

11. Wille, H., and Molgaard, I. Giant papillary conjunctivitis in connection with corneal scleral supramid (nylon) suture knots. *Acta Ophthalmol.*, 62:75–83, 1984.

12. Friedman, T., Friedman, Z., and Neuman, E. Giant papillary conjunctivitis following cataract extraction. *Ann. Ophthalmol.*, 16:50–52, 1984.

13. Sugar, A., and Meyer, R. F. Giant papillary conjunctivitis after keratoplasty. *Am. J. Ophthalmol.*, 91:239–242, 1981.

14. Korb, D. R., Allansmith, M. R., Greiner, J. V., et al. Prevalance of conjunctival changes in wearers of hard contact lenses. *Am. J. Ophthalmol.*, 90:336–341, 1980.

15. Allansmith, M. R., Greiner, J. V., and Baird, R. S. Number of inflammatory cells in the normal conjunctiva. *Am. J. Ophthalmol.*, 85:250–259, 1978.

16. Allansmith, M. R., Greiner, J. V., and Baird, R. S. Number and type of inflammatory cells in conjunctiva of asymptomatic contact lens wearers. *Am. J. Ophthalmol.*, 87:171–174, 1979.

17. Allansmith, M. R., Korb, D. R., and Greiner, J. V. Giant papillary conjunctivitis induced by hard or soft contact lens wear: Quantitative histology. *Ophthalmology (Rochester)*, 85:766–778, 1978.

18. Allansmith, M. R., Baird, R. S., and Greiner, J. V. Vernal conjunctivitis and contact lens associated giant papillary conjunctivitis compared and contrasted. *Am. J. Ophthalmol.*, 87:544–555, 1979.

19. Henriquez, A. S., and Allansmith, M. R. Russell bodies in contact lens associated giant papillary conjunctivitis. *Arch. Ophthalmol.*, 97:473–478, 1979.

20. Donshik, P. C., and Ballow, M. Tear immunoglobulins in giant papillary conjunctivitis induced by contact lens. *Am. J. Ophthalmol.*, 96:460–466, 1983.

21. Ballow, M., Donshik, P. C., and Mendelson, L. Complement proteins and C3 anaphylatoxin in tears of patients with conjunctivitis. *J Allergy Clin. Immunol.*, 76:473–476, 1985.

22. Ballow, M., Donshik, P., Rapacz, P., and Samartino, L. Tear lactoferrin levels in patients with external inflammatory ocular disease. *Invest. Ophthalmol.*, 28:543–545, 1987.

23. Donshik, P. C., Tedesco, J., Rapacz, P., and Ballow, M. Tear lysozyme levels in patients with contact lens induced giant papillary conjunctivitis and vernal conjunctivitis. *Invest. Ophthalmol.*, 28(3):38, 1987.

24. Fowler, S. A., Greiner, J. V., and Allansmith, M. R. Soft contact lenses from patients with giant papillary conjunctivitis. *Am. J. Ophthalmol.*, 88:1056–1066, 1979.

25. Ballow, M., Rapacz, P., Maenza, R., Yamase, H., and Donshik, P. C. An animal model for contact lens induced giant papillary conjunctivitis. *Invest. Ophthalmol.*, 28(3):39, 1987.

26. Fowler, S. A., and Allansmith, M. R. The effect of cleaning contact lenses. *Arch. Ophthalmol.*, 99:1382–1386, 1981.

27. Donshik, P. C., Ballow, M., Luistro, A., and Samartino, L. Treatment of contact lens induced giant papillary conjunctivitis. *CLAO J.*, 10:346–350, 1984.

28. Foreman, S. L., and Garland, L. G. Cromoglycate and other antiallergic drugs: A possible mechanism of action. *Br. Med. J.*, 1:820–821, 1976.

29. Friday, G. A., Biglaw, A. W., and Hiles, D. A. Treatment of ragweed allergic conjunctivitis with cromolyn 4% ophthalmic solution. *Am. J. Ophthalmol.*, 95:169–174, 1983.

30. Collum, L. M. T., Cassidy, H. P., and Benedict-Smith, A. Disodium crologlycate in vernal and allergic keratoconjunctivitis. *Ir. Med. J.*, 74:14–18, 1981.

31. Foster, C. S., and Duncan, J. Randomized clinical trial of topically administered cromolyn sodium for vernal keratoconjunctivitis. *Am. J. Ophthalmol.*, 90:175–181, 1980.

32. Meisler, D. M., Berzin, V. J., Krachmer, J. H., et al. Cromolyn treatment of giant papillary conjunctivitis. *Arch. Ophthalmology*, 100:1608–1610, 1987.

11
FUTURE DEVELOPMENTS IN RIGID GAS-PERMEABLE CONTACT LENSES

During the past several years, the contact lens practitioner has witnessed a revolution in the development of rigid gas-permeable lens materials. In the early 1970s the introduction of cellulose acetate butyrate (CAB) lenses seemed like a major advance in that they provided a slight degree of oxygen permeability. With the availability of the first silicone acrylate lenses in Canada in 1976, the revolution appeared to be in full swing, since these lenses virtually eliminated the classic PMMA central corneal clouding hypoxic response (Fig. 11.1).

Today, currently available rigid gas-permeable lens materials allow as much (and, in many cases, more) oxygen transmissibility as extended-wear hydrogel lenses. One might wonder if the revolution is reaching an endpoint or at least slowing down somewhat. However, as each new milestone is achieved, it brings with it a host of new challenges.

IDEAL CHARACTERISTICS OF RIGID GAS-PERMEABLE LENS MATERIALS

In a broad sense, the ideal lens material will provide excellent corneal and conjunctival health, consistently clear visual acuity, predictable fitting characteristics, and reproducible manufacturing. To fully understand what will be necessary to achieve these goals, we must examine specific clinical performance characteristics:

PHYSIOLOGICAL RESPONSE

With the advent and continuing development of rigid gas-permeable materials, much attention has been focused on the measurement of oxygen permeability (D_k). Unfortunately, in the

Fig. 11.1 *Central corneal clouding with hypoxic response with PMMA lens.*

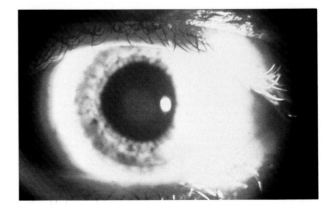

marketplace, through implication and not scientific fact, it is stated that D_k measurements are

1. directly correlated with the corneal response,
2. directly correlated with patient success,
3. directly correlated with patient comfort, and
4. a substitute for an appropriate lens design and fitting.

Clinically, this is just not the case. Oxygen permeability is a critically important characteristic in determining the corneal response to lens wear but does not tell the entire story. Oxygen transmissibility D_k/L, which factors in lens thickness, is a much better guide to corneal response. However, as lens materials approach the permeability of the tear film (D_k 78) itself, even D_k/L loses its accuracy as a predictor of the corneal response as a result of the boundary layer effect (1). The only true way to understand the physiological response is to observe it (2). Clinical manifestations of relative corneal hypoxia include the following: increases in corneal thickness with or without striae (pachometry); epithelial microcysts; a decrease in stromal pH due to lactic acid accumulation; epithelial thickening; stromal thickening; and endothelial polymegathism and pleomorphism.

Ideally, we would like to create a lens material that has no physiological impact. That is, even by using extremely sensitive measurements of hypoxic response (pachometry, stromal pH, and morphometric analysis of the corneal endothelium), we must achieve a level of oxygen flux to the cornea that causes minimal, if any, disturbance.

To produce virtually no change in corneal thickness under daily wear conditions, a lens must provide an equivalent oxygen percentage (EOP) of no less than 10% (3). Theoretically, this requires a D_k/L of approximately 18–20 (Table 11.1). Clinically,

TABLE 11.1
D_k VALUES

Material Name	D_k (Stated as per Uncorrected Fatt) at 35°C	Recommended Thickness at −3.00 diopters	D_k/L
The Boston Lens IV	28	0.15	18.7
Optacryl K	31	0.16	20.1
Paraperm 02+	39	0.16	24.3

this is quite accurate and may be readily achieved by several currently available lens materials. However, to achieve a near-zero increase above the 4–5% baseline physiological response of corneal thickening during overnight wear is a different matter. Theoretically, this requires a D_k/L of 75 (Ref. 4) and is not obtained by any commercially available rigid gas-permeable or hydrogel material at this time. Even the silicone acrylate lenses which have received FDA approval or are pending approval for overnight wear do not provide this level of oxygenation. Several manufacturers have marketed, or plan to market, lenses in the near future which are closer to this goal than ever before (Table 11.2).

As mentioned earlier, the true prognostic value of D_k is limited by the boundary layer effect as the D_k approaches 70. The only accurate way to assess overnight swelling response is to measure it.

Polse et al. (5) and Andrasko (6) have confirmed the overnight swelling response with The Boston Equalens (TBEQ) to be 5.6% and 6.6% above baseline, respectively.

Thus, we are rapidly approaching an oxygen flux level with rigid gas-permeable lens materials that will cause only minimal, if any, increase in corneal thickness on overnight wear.

Another "ideal" measurement of physiological response is a change in stromal pH to indicate lactic acid accumulation. Bonanno and Polse (7) have reported on a technique for measuring stromal pH. Their preliminary report indicates that the pure fluoropolymer (3M) and the Boston experimental fluoro-silicone acrylate lenses are quite close to achieving a physiologic state.

TABLE 11.2
HIGHER-D_k-VALUE LENSES

Material Name	Material Type	Dk (Stated as per Uncorrected Fatt at 35°C)	Recommended Thickness at −3.00D	D_k/L
The Boston Lens IV	Silicone acrylate	28	0.15	18.7
Optacryl K	Silicone acrylate	31	0.15	20.1
Paraperm EW	Silicone acrylate	56	0.18	31.1
Optacryl EXT	Silicone acrylate	59	0.18	32.7
Optacryl Z	Silicone acrylate	84	0.18	46.7
The Boston Equalens	Fluorosilicone acrylate	71	0.15	47.3
Fluoroperm	Fluorosilicone acrylate	97	0.19	51.0
Quantum 1	Fluorosilicone acrylate	92	0.17	54.1
3M Fluoropolymer	Fluoropolymer	170	0.22	77.3
Quantum II	Fluorosilicone acrylate	210	0.18	116.6
The Boston Equalens II	Fluorosilicone acrylate	203	0.16	126.9

Lastly, alterations in endothelial morphology give us further information as to the long-term corneal tolerance to lens wear. Certainly a goal for material manufacturers and lens designers is to develop lenses that cause no alterations in endothelial morphology when worn for daily as well as overnight wear (Figs. 11.2 and 11.3). Preliminary 6-month reports from Polse indicate a 5% polymegathism with TBEQ when worn for extended wear (5). Preliminary 6-month reports by Schoessler indicate similar results.

The only lenses reported to produce no morphological changes in the corneal endothelium have been silicone elastomer (8). It has been widely written that the etiology of altered endothelial morphology is directly related to hypoxia and lactic acid production. As such, the degree of endothelial polymegathism and pleomorphism that will be induced may be viewed as follows:

PMMA > Hydrogels worn for extended-wear > Daily-wear hydrogels
Low-oxygen-flux RGPs (D_k/L 7–15)RGPs > Medium-oxygen-flux RGPs
(D_k/L 20–40) > High-oxygen-flux RGPs (D_k/L > 40)

In summary, with the future availability of high-oxygen-flux fluorosilicone acrylates and other fluoropolymers, the physiological response to lens wear will approach having no lens on the eye.

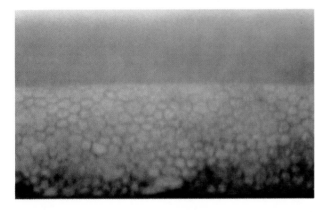

Fig. 11.2 *Normal endothelium.*

Fig. 11.3 *Marked polymegathism and pleomorphism. (Courtesy of John Schoessler, Ph.D., Ohio State University.)*

DEPOSIT RESISTANCE AND IN-EYE WETTABILITY

If a contact lens is to be worn safely and effectively for prolonged periods, it must resist the formation of surface deposits; otherwise the cornea and conjunctiva will suffer mechanical and/or immunological compromise. Clinical manifestations of inadequate deposit resistance and resultant lens coating include: giant papillary conjunctivitis; lens awareness and irritation; poor surface wetting and dessication; lens filming with associated blurred vision; superficial punctate keratitis (SPK); and, in extreme cases, toxic keratopathy. *Surface hazing* refers to the drying of the contact lens surface with the adhesion of mucous debris. It may occur most frequently with silicone acrylate lenses and, to a much smaller extent, with the fluorosilicone acrylate materials (Figs. 11.4 and 11.5).

Deposit resistance in current and future materials will depend on three principal factors:

1. care regimen;
2. surface quality produced during manufacturing; and
3. specific polymer properties.

THE LENS CARE REGIMEN

Lens hygiene plays a key role in the management of deposits on gas-permeable lens surfaces. If a lens is not cleaned thoroughly, the remaining debris which is hydrophobic will tend to attract even more debris via a mechanism of hydrophobic interaction.

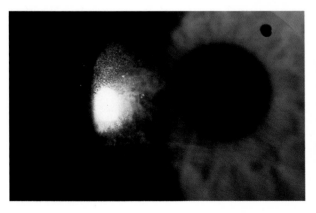

Fig. 11.4 *Relative surface-hazing phenomenon on Boston IV lens.*

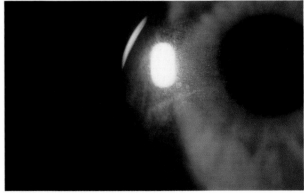

Fig. 11.5 *Relative surface-hazing phenomenon on Equalens.*

Unfortunately, the tenacity with which proteinaceous material adsorbs onto silicone acrylate lens surfaces is extreme. Unlike PMMA surfaces, which are nonreactive, silicone acrylate surfaces are highly reactive. The deposit tenacity occurs because surface deposits on silicone acrylate lenses tend to be the result of specific chemical interactions, namely, hydrophobic interaction and electrostatic interaction (Fig. 11.6).

To effectively clean these surfaces requires specially formulated friction-enhanced surfactant cleaners which first mechanically break the bonds between the lens and the absorbed debris. Only then will it be possible to solubilize and rinse away the deposited material. Even with the use of abrasive cleaners, certain patients may not achieve truly clean, protein-free lens surfaces. For those patients, the use of proteolytic enzymes is indicated. Until the time arrives when the polymer composition reduces the stubbornness of the deposit, these measures will be necessary.

SURFACE QUALITY

Another factor in predisposing all types of lenses to surface deposition is the inadequate preparation of high-quality surfaces. As materials become more sophisticated, they often become considerably more difficult to manufacture. Techniques, procedures, and equipment that are quite adequate for fabricating low(10–20)- and medium(20–40)-D_k materials may not be ad-

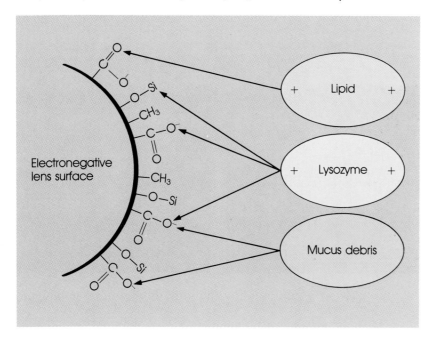

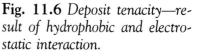

Fig. 11.6 *Deposit tenacity—result of hydrophobic and electrostatic interaction.*

equate for high-D_k materials, particularly fluorinated materials. As a result, lens surfaces may be torn, burned, or heated to a point where the plastic actually begins to flow. (Figs. 11.7 and 11.8). This ultimately compromises the surface and potentially interferes with its chemical affinity for tear debris. Even the most deposit-resistant lens material will coat profoundly if not prepared properly.

Certainly, if material development is to continue, the state-of-the-art in manufacturing procedures must lead the way to ensure the utmost performance of the material.

POLYMER PROPERTIES

As we search for high levels of oxygen permeability to achieve safe overnight wear, there is a need to understand the limitations of materials. All silicon-containing rigid gas-permeable materials are prone to deposition by tear components. This affinity for denatured proteins is dependent on the polymer composition but generally will increase as a function of the silicon content. Polymer scientists known that there is no "free ride" in polymer formulations. This is especially true of silicone acrylate materials. The siloxane moiety (silicon-containing monomer) is unequaled in its oxygen transmission capabilities. However, incorporating enough siloxane to achieve the oxygen flux levels necessary for safe overnight wear brings with it the stigma of reducing wettability, increasing the adhesion of mucous debris, and accelerating the formation of surface deposits. The undesirable properties can be somewhat managed by the judicious incorporation of wetting agents. However, the maximum level of wetting components is limited by the tendency of these components to ad-

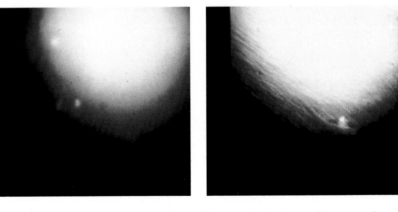

Fig. 11.7 *Normal high quality lens surface.* **Fig. 11.8** *Burned lens surface.*

versely affect dimensional stability. For this reason, silicone acrylate lens materials will have only limited application in the future.

As can be seen from Table 11.1, a major development in progress is the incorporation of fluorine into the next generation of rigid gas-permeable lens materials. Two specific trends will be evident in fluorinated materials development. First, a group of materials similar to current material with regard to fitting, manufacturing, and optical characteristics will evolve. These materials, the fluorosilicone acrylates, will fully exploit the oxygen transmission capabilities of the siloxane moiety but, through the incorporation of the element fluorine, will have markedly improved in-eye wettability and deposit resistance (Figs. 11.9 and 11.10). The addition of fluorinated monomers has a profound effect on the surface of the polymer and, as such, offsets the undesirable hydrophobic characteristics brought on by significant increases in siloxane content. What is achieved is a wet lens surface that, unlike ordinary silicone acrylates, does not promote a firm binding of proteinaceous tear constituents and mucuous debris. That is, even when deposition does occur, the deposits are loosely bound and are removed by the simple squeegee action of the blinking eyelid. This is fundamentally different than what is found with silicone acrylate lenses (9) and is of significant benefit to patient comfort as well as corneal and conjunctival health.

The second type of fluorinated material, the pure fluoropolymer, will require revisions in fitting techniques, manufacturing procedures, and optical performance latitude. However, it has been reported to provide exceptional physiological response and

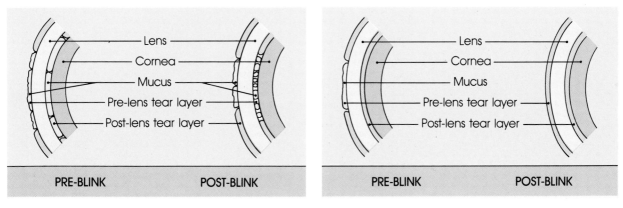

Fig. 11.9 *Silicone acrylate mucous binding.* Fig. 11.10 *Fluorosilicone mucous binding.*

deposit resistance (10). Both types of material will approach virtually no physiologic impact as mentioned earlier but, in addition, will afford a surface biocompatibility with the preocular tear film, corneal surface, and conjunctiva unapproached by any previous materials.

FLEXURAL RESISTANCE

In our search for the "ideal" future lens material, let's not lose sight of the fact that rigid gas-permeable lenses are worn predominantly for the cosmetic correction of refractive errors. Future developments must provide materials that can be manufactured in a wide range of optical corrections and back-surface geometries in order to allow successful management of all ametropias and corneal topographies. In addition, new materials must be sufficiently rigid so that regular and irregular topographies do not transmit unwanted cylindrical correction into the lens refractive power. Lens flexure is a clinical performance characteristic that can be easily compromised as we increase the silicon content in the polymer formulation. That is, once again, as we attempt to reach high oxygen-flux levels in ordinary silicone acrylate lenses by increasing the silicone content, we can easily lose the flexural resistance, and thus the optical performance, of the lens. Clinicians and manufacturers often remedy flexibility in these polymers by increasing lens thickness to "stiffen" the final lens form. However, this is quite counterproductive in the quest for greater oxygen transmissibility (D_k/L).

Clinicians should be suspect of materials not capable of affording good-quality optical correction in astigmatic patients. Whereas poor optical correction is annoying to the patient, excessively flexible materials may undergo a stress relief phenomenon due to repeated on-eye flexure. This has been manifested clinically as surface crazing (Figs. 11.11 and 11.12). Initially, crazing looks like deep scratches or layered deposition but cannot be removed by lens polishing. Upon close inspection, these fissures can be observed in the polymer matrix. If the patient is allowed to continue to wear crazed lenses, the phenomenon may progress to fine surface cracks which, on the anterior surface, will predispose to deposit formation and, on the posterior surface, may cause corneal abrasions(11).

Future materials, then, should not be so soft, due to high silicon or fluorine contents, that vision correction is compromised. This will be achieved through the incorporating of novel cross-linking agents or other monomers to stiffen, without making brittle, the polymer backbone. As new materials are developed, the clinician should draw on the worldwide experience so that he/she will "get a feel" for which plastics are too soft to give good visual acuity, which plastics are too brittle to be durable during patient handling, and which may have idiosyncrasies such as crazing.

DIMENSIONAL STABILITY

The dimensional stability of future generations of rigid gas-permeable materials will depend on the lens manufacturing process and the individual polymer formulation.

Along with dimensional changes related to hydration are changes that occur due to differential force being applied to the lens as a result of a single-radius (spherical) posterior surface being worn on a moderately to highly toric cornea. Ultimately, after months of wearing, it is not uncommon or unexpected for the posterior surface to show some degree of induced toricity relative to the degree of corneal toricity. This "warpage" occurs with PMMA occasionally but occurs to a more noticeable extent with increasing levels of oxygen permeability. Probably this reflects a lesser material hardness and/or modulus as a function of increased silicon or fluorine content. Small amounts of induced back-surface toricity rarely affect vision. The clinician need *not* be concerned about induced back-surface toricity unless there is either a compromise in subjective visual acuity or enough topographical change to significantly alter the fitting relationship.

If clinicians accept slight degrees of induced toricity as one of the small trade-offs of enhanced permeability and wettabil-

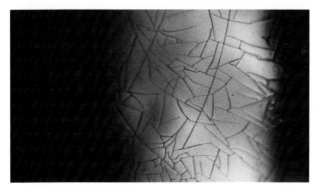

Fig. 11.11 *High-D_k silicone acrylate lens crazing.*

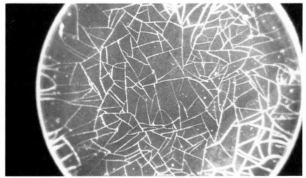

Fig. 11.12 *High-D_k silicone acrylate lens crazing.*

ity/deposit resistance brought about by greater silicon and fluorine content, respectively, the clinical performance of future materials will be quite an impressive breakthrough.

The future of rigid gas-permeable materials undoubtedly seems to be very close to achieving our goals of corneal and conjunctival health and excellent visual acuity through the development of fluorinated materials. However, as we approach the point of being physiologically undetectable and extremely surface biocompatible, we also encounter a new set of fitting characteristics. That is, even state-of-the-art materials need to be well fit to be successful. For this reason, future materials will, out of necessity, have to be combined with more refined geometries to achieve a *design compatibility*.

If patients and practitioners are to realize the overall benefits of rigid gas-permeable lenses relative to hydrogel lenses, two major factors need to be overcome. These are: (i) the comfort upon insertion and during initial adaptation; and (ii) a system of rapid, reproducible fitting.

Comfort of rigid gas-permeable lenses is a function of the material biocompatibility (permeability, in-eye wettability, resistance to deposit formation/mucous adhesion, and coefficient of friction), an even tear-film profile creating a zero pressure gradient of lens–cornea baring (Figs. 11.13 and 11.14), and an optimal edge clearance.

Fig. 11.13 *Even tear-film profile with zero pressure gradient of lens cornea baring and optimal edge lift.*

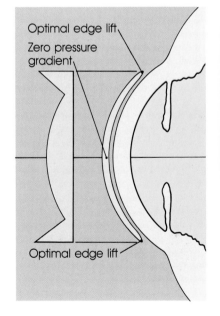

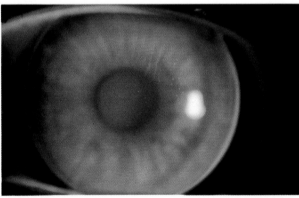

Fig. 11.14 *Even tear-film profile with zero pressure gradient of lens cornea baring and optimal edge lift.*

The material biocompatibility has been addressed at length. From all indications, fluorinated materials will make this factor a non-issue.

Achieving a zero pressure gradient of lens–cornea baring can vary from being relatively easy to virtually impossible on toric or post-surgical eyes (Fig. 11.15). Even though a midperipheral baring area (Fig. 11.16) may appear relatively small and of no consequence when viewed in a static position, lens decentration during the blink will create a high-pressure seal-off on the cornea. This will be particularly true of the future high-D_k lens materials that will be prone to compression flexure during the blink cycle. Thus, obtaining an even tear-film distribution free of baring zones is critically important to achieving comfort.

The experienced fitter may, through painstaking time and effort, achieve this by fully exploiting lens geometry relationships in trial fitting, taking peripheral corneal measurements or photographs, or by using a computer-assisted tear-film model. Practically speaking, it is desirable to take the knowledge obtained by topographic analysis of a widespread population and model a posterior surface geometry that approximates the corneal shape.

If we consider that the central cornea is an ellipse of eccentricity approximately 0.4 (Ref. 12) and gradually flattens in the periphery, it is easy to understand why trying to achieve an even

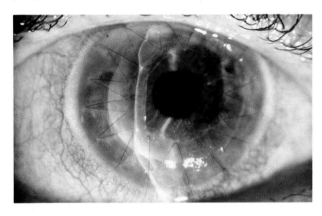

Fig. 11.15 *Irregular corneal topography secondary to post-penetrating-keratoplasty.*

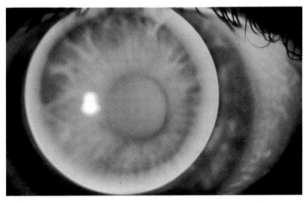

Fig. 11.16 *Midperipheral baring.*

tear-film distribution by placing spherical posterior-surface lenses on such a shape is quite difficult. At best, an even alignment is only possible within the central 5–6 mm. This still leaves probable baring areas in the midperiphery. If the fitter reduces the sagittal depth relationship by decreasing the optic zone or diameter or by increasing the base curve radius, it may be possible to minimize midperipheral baring. However, these parameter changes can adversely alter the centration and/or central lens–cornea relationship.

It is well understood that placing intermediate and peripheral curves of progressively flatter radius on the posterior lens surface is necessary to provide clearance in the lens periphery. By using multicurve blended spherical lenses, we are attempting to approximate the progressive flattening in the corneal midperiphery and periphery. Because laboratory fabrication of such designs is performed in part by hand, human error is inevitable. Thus, it is possible, but time consuming and somewhat complex, to achieve reproducible consistent fitting characteristics when using spherical multicurve lenses.

Logic tells us that to obtain the even tear-film profile and zero pressure gradient for optimum comfort, we need to create a lens geometry that approximates the relatively low eccentricity of the central cornea ($e \approx 0.4$) in the optic zone area as well as approximate the hyperboloid shape ($e > 1.0$) of the peripheral cornea.

Obviously, then, a minimum of two different eccentricities is necessary. Also of significant importance is that the two curves be computed so that their junction occurs at the point at which their rate of change is equal.

This creates a continuously changing junctionless back-surface curvature. Blending or hand-grinding the back surface will become totally unnecessary. By combining these computations with an axis-driven computer numerical control lathe, it will be possible to reproducibly generate the biaspheric design with a high degree of precision.

In addition, by using aspheric curvatures, it is possible to significantly reduce the amount of edge lift necessary. This results in physiologically better fitting, as well as markedly improved patient comfort, and allows large degrees of corneal astigmatism to be fitted compared to spherical multicurve designs (Figs. 11.17–19). In fact, Z values for aspheric lenses are approximately 50–85% less than their multicurve counterparts (13) (Table 11.3).

For these reasons, utilizing aspheric technology for lens designs readily permits us to obtain a design compatibility with future materials. In doing so, rapid reproducible fitting and comfort approaching that of hydrogel lenses within minutes of insertion will be achieved.

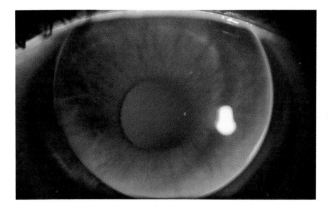

Fig. 11.17 *Biaspheric design on 1.00-diopter corneal cylinder.*

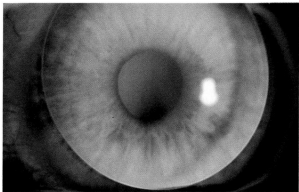

Fig. 11.18 *Biaspheric design on 3.00-diopter corneal cylinder.*

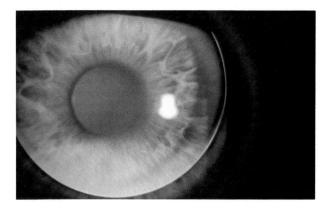

Fig. 11.19 *Biaspheric design on 5.00-diopter corneal cylinder.*

TABLE 11.3
COMPARISON OF Z VALUES FOR
MULTICURVE SPHERICAL LENSES
AND ELLIPTICAL LENSES

Diameter	Recommended Multicurve Z Values for Lenses Spherical	Z Values for $e \approx 0.4$ Elliptical Lenses
8.80	0.095–1.05	0.016–0.030
9.30	0.098–0.111	0.020–0.041
9.80	0.102–0.103	0.025–0.053

REFERENCES

1. Brennan, N. A., Efron, N., and Holden, B. A. Further developments in the HGP Dk debate. *Int. Eyecare,* 2(10):xx, 1986.

2. Mandell, R. A. Contact lens transmissibility and corneal swelling. Presented at the American Academy of Optometry, Toronto, Ontario, December 1986.

3. Holden, B. A., Sweeny, D. F., and Sanderson, G. The minimum pre-corneal oxygen tension to avoid corneal edema. *Invest. Ophthalmol. Vis. Sci.,* 25:476, 1984.

4. O'Neal, M. R., Polse, K. A., and Sarver, M. D. Corneal response to rigid and hydrogel lenses during eye closure. *Invest. Ophthalmol. Vis. Sci.,* 25:837–842, 1984.

5. Polse, K. A., Sarver, M. D., Rivera, R. K., and Bonanno, J. Ocular and visual effects of hard gas permeable lens extended wear. Presented at the American Academy of Optometry, Toronto, Ontario, December 1986.

6. Andrasko, G. A. Corneal swelling and deswelling comparisons after HGP and soft extended wear. Presented at the American Academy of Optometry, Toronto, Ontario, December 1986.

7. Bonanno, J. A., and Polse, K. A. Effect of contact lens wear on stromal pH. Presented at the American Academy of Optometry, Toronto, Ontario, December 1986.

8. Schoessler, J. P., Barr, J. T., and Freson, D. R. Corneal endothelial observations of silicone elastomer contact lens wearers. *Int. Contact Lens Clinic* 11(6):337 (1984).

9. Gleason, W. J. and Doane, M. G. Contact angle vs. in vivo lens wetting evaluation. Presented at the American Academy of Optometry, Toronto, Ontario, December 1986.

10. Holden, B. A., LaHood, D., Sweeny, D. H., Schnider, C., and Kenyon, E. The critical oxygen levels required with rigid gas permeable lenses required to avoid adverse physiological effect on extended wear. Presented at the American Academy of Optometry, Toronto, Ontario, December 1986.

11. Grohe, R. M. Comparative surface hazing of silicone acrylate and fluorosilicone acrylate copolymer contact lenses. Presented at the American Academy of Optometry, Toronto, Ontario, December 1986.

12. Kiely, P. M., Smith, G., and Carney, L. C. Meridional variations in corneal shape. *Am. J. Optom. Physiol. Opt.,* 61:10, 619–626 (1981).

13. Grant, R. The elliptical fitting philosophy; hard gas permeable lenses. *The Optician,* February 7, 1986.

INDEX